Predicting Successful Hospital Mergers and Acquisitions
A Financial and Marketing Analytical Tool

Predicting Successful Hospital Mergers and Acquisitions

A Financial and Marketing Analytical Tool

David P. Angrisani, PhD, CPA
Robert L. Goldman, PhD

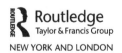

Routledge
Taylor & Francis Group

NEW YORK AND LONDON

First published 1997 by Haworth Press, Inc.

Published 2010 by Routledge
711 Third Avenue, New York, NY 10017
2 Park Square, Milton Park, Abingdon, Oxon, OX14 4RN

Routledge is an imprint of the Taylor & Francis Group, an informa business

Cover design by Marylouise E. Doyle.

Library of Congress Cataloging-in-Publication Data

Angrisani, David P.
  Predicting successful hospital mergers and acquisitions : a financial and marketing analytical tool / by David P. Angrisani, Robert L. Goldman.
    p.   cm.
  Includes bibliographical references and index.
  ISBN 0-7890-0057-1 (hard : alk. paper)
  1. Hospital mergers. I. Goldman, Robert, 1937-   . II. Title. [DNLM: 1. Health Facility Merger–economics. 2. Financial Management, Hospital. 3. Hospital Restructuring–economics. 4. Models, Economic. WX 157 A588p 1997]
RA971.A794 1997
362.1'1'0681–dc20
DNLM/DLC
for Library of Congress   96-24638
                                                          0-7890-0182-9   CIP

Publisher's Note
The publisher has gone to great lengths to ensure the quality of this reprint but points out that some imperfections in the original may be apparent.

CONTENTS

ABOUT THE AUTHORS

David P. Angrisani, PhD, CPA, is Associate Professor of Business and Director of the MBA degree program at Holy Names College in Oakland, California. He is also Adjunct Professor at the University of California, Berkeley, where he teaches financial accounting. Dr. Angrisani has over eighteen years of experience teaching and is a financial and tax consultant for various business organizations.

Robert L. Goldman, PhD, is Vice President of Health Care Management for Centerex Corporation in San Francisco, California, and Academic Dean of the International University of America. He has over twenty-five years health care management and marketing experience as both a consultant and an executive in the United States and Eastern Europe. A nationally recognized speaker, Dr. Goldman has published numerous articles on health care marketing and management, health care marketing ethics, and the development of private health care in formerly socialist countries. He also consults with health care and health care-related organizations that desire to enter the Japanese market.

ABOUT THE AUTHORS

Chapter 1

What This Book Will Do for You: Introduction

This book is designed as a tool that hospital and hospital system executives can use to determine the potential success of a merger or acquisition within the nonfederal hospital sector. We did not examine other types of mergers involving hospitals, such as long-term care facilities or physician groups. Particular emphasis needs to be given to the effect of managed care in future merger analysis.

We believe that there are three factors that must be considered when reviewing a prospective merger or acquisition: (1) the financial viability of the new unit; (2) the positive or negative effects on the marketing efforts of this entity; and (3) its potential for increased operational success and efficiency. Each element is analyzed and reviewed with regard to its relation to the others.

We have analyzed data on all mergers and acquisitions of California hospitals between 1982 and 1992. There was a total of 29 mergers during that period. (Note: Data on mergers within the Kaiser system were not available.) We first analyzed the data to determine *which* hospitals were potential candidates for mergers.

Data from five years prior and up to three years after merger or acquisition are compared. We also attempted to compare these hospitals with hospitals of similar revenue, size, and type of location that had not merged or acquired another hospital.

From this data we attempted to develop a model that would predict a merger candidate. We found seven significant financial variables that would discriminate between merger candidates and nontargeted hospitals.

We found that the model was successful in predicting merger or acquisition targets. The success rate varied from 55 percent to 93 percent. The variance of the results was due to the age of the data. That is, predictions based on data from five years before a merger were less accurate while data from one year before a merger permitted extremely accurate predictions.

We determined seven significant financial variables from one year prior to the merger or acquisition for the buying hospital and the new organization. Examining these seven variables, we concluded that the new organization was negatively impacted by the merger or acquisition. However, these variables could not predict the success or failure of the new organization.

Still, we attempted to predict the potential for success of the new organizations with this model. We found that our analysis of financial data alone, *based on a single financial ratio*, could predict failure with a high degree of accuracy and success with less precision.

Thus, we see two potential conclusions from this work. First, that if the executives studying the potential merger or acquisition reviewed these variables, they would have a fairly good idea whether or not the new organization would be better or worse off financially than the old organization initiating the transaction. Second, we can conclude that these mergers are taking place because of nonfinancial factors that *offset the negative financial impact in the long run*. If not, then these very talented and intelligent executives made bad decisions for their organizations. To conclude, we review what has happened with as many of these mergers and acquisitions as possible.

MERGERS AND ACQUISITIONS
AS A GROWTH STRATEGY

There are four possibilities for growth as seen in Figure 1.1: market penetration, market development, product/service development, and diversification. A review of the definitions of these terms, as stated in one of the popular marketing textbooks, will aid our discussion.

Market penetration is trying to increase sales of a firm's present products in its present markets—probably through a more aggressive marketing mix. The firm may try to increase the customers' rate of use or attract competitors' customers or current nonusers. For ex-

FIGURE 1.1. Four Possibilities for Growth

	Present Products	New Products
Present markets	Market penetration	Product development
New markets	Market development	Diversification

Source: E. Jerome McCarthy and William D. Perreault Jr., *Basic Marketing*, 10th edition. Homewood, IL: Irwin, p. 66.

ample, Coca-Cola has increased advertising to encourage people to take a morning Coke break instead of a coffee break and to switch from Diet Pepsi to Diet Coke.

New promotion appeals alone may not be effective. A firm may need to add more stores in present areas for greater customer convenience. Short-term price cuts or coupon offers may help. For example, AT&T has increased advertising and offered special discounts to encourage customers to choose AT&T over other long-distance telephone services.

Obviously, effective planning is aided by a real understanding of why some people are buying now and what will motivate them to shift brands, buy more, begin purchasing, or resume buying.

Market development is trying to increase sales by selling present products in new markets. This may only involve advertising in different media to reach new target customers. Or it may mean adding channels of distribution or new stores in new areas. For example, McDonald's is reaching new customers by opening outlets in airports, office buildings, zoos, casinos, hospitals, and military bases. And the franchise is rapidly expanding into international markets with outlets in places such as Brazil, Hong Kong, and Australia.

Market development may also involve a search for new uses for a product, as when Lipton provides recipes that indicate how to use its dry soup mixes to make party dips.

Product development is offering new or improved products for present markets. Here, the firm should know the market's needs; it may see ways of adding or modifying product features, creating several quality levels, or adding more types or sizes to better satisfy them. Computer software firms such as Microsoft boost sales by introducing new versions of popular programs. Microsoft has also developed other types of new products for its customers. It now sells computer books and even computer hardware.

Diversification is moving into totally different lines of business—which may include entirely unfamiliar products, markets, or even levels in the production-marketing system. Until recently, Sony was strictly a producer of electronic equipment. With its purchase of CBS records, it has expanded into producing music—and it is considering other moves that will take it further yet from its traditional business.[1]

Mergers or acquisitions may be used within each of these strategies. For example, by acquiring a hospital within your current market, you may increase market share to help customers, such as HMOs, identify your organization as the one that they want to do business with.

By adding hospitals in a market that you have not entered, you have the opportunity to develop that market for your brand. Often, expansion into new markets is accomplished by buying "fire sale" units and restoring them to health. Of course, this can be accomplished in your current markets or in new markets.

An acute care hospital organization that buys long-term care, rehabilitation, and/or psychiatric units is moving into product development strategy. To differentiate this strategy from diversification, you can see that the additions listed in the definition are still within the provision of hospital-type care. Acquiring a drug wholesaler would be more akin to diversification.

While the correct nomenclature is not important, the concept that an organization can increase sales and improve revenues through the acquisition of or merger with other organizations is important. Because few new markets are available for hospitals and because competition is increasing, the merger and/or acquisition route may be the only one available for organizations that want to grow.

We want to caution you about one facet of using an acquisition strategy to capture market share. That is, there are regulatory restrictions that must be considered. We will review the current published opinions. However, only legal counsel can give you a definitive answer.

MERGERS AND ACQUISITIONS
AS A DEFENSIVE STRATEGY

Another organization seems to be interested in a market that you have had your eye on for some time. You do not see its value within your current strategic plan. However, you do have plans for it in the future. By acquiring a unit within this market you can forestall the move that your competition seems to want to make.

There is danger in this strategy. You may find that your acquisition costs are only the first installment that you will have to pay. If the new market needs development, you may find that it will take years for the unit to break even.

To Succeed, Both Financial and Marketing Aspects
Must Be Considered

To remain competitive and efficient in the current managed care environment, hospitals and other health service institutions must continually reassess their market positions. This may mean eliminating or otherwise modifying services to cut costs.

The other option is to increase revenues. If it is possible to acquire a new unit that permits economies of scale or offers other incentives, it is wiser—in the long run—to attempt to build up an organization instead of trying to downsize since there are limits to the savings that you can obtain as your system or hospital shrinks.

Operational Aspects Affect the Success of a Merger
or Acquisition

All too often a unit may look ideal for acquisition or merger only to find that the financial and marketing elements were fine but that there were operational aspects that were not considered.

The merger of medical staffs has caused problems in even the smoothest transition. A warning sign of potential trouble is when the two units to be merged are geographically close together. This may indicate that the staffs chose not to work cooperatively because of job insecurity.

Redundant employees need to be released with a minimum of trauma. If one hospital is unionized and the other is not, you can expect some difficult problems. Finding a method to retain the best employees–without raising issues such as age discrimination–will take much of your time. Of course, the differences between the utility of the physical plants will also be of major concern.

Differing corporate cultures and community images may become apparent. You will see that caution is essential when analyzing the factors and applying cost/benefit ratios to them.

Quality is an important factor that may be affected by the formation of a new entity. We will discuss operational quality and customer service quality. Quality goes beyond numbers and it goes below the surface. Quality is not merely what people will accept, nor is a set of statistical norms that can be reported to the Board on a quarterly basis.

In discussing what level of quality you need to achieve to compete in the managed care environment, we also discuss centers of excellence. We believe that managed care organizations will contract only with true regional centers that offer unique services at a level of quality acceptable to knowledgeable consumers. "Me Too" centers may actually cost you money if they are included in your capitation payment. We also discuss nonmanaged centers that can be very profitable and attract patients.

REFERENCE NOTE

1. E. Jerome McCarthy and William D. Perreault Jr., *Basic Marketing*, 10th edition, Homewood, IL: Irwin, 1990, 65-67.

Chapter 2

Review of Previous Studies

EARLY STUDIES

The use of financial data and accounting numbers to analyze firms and their performance dates back almost 100 years. The accounting and finance literature is abundant with studies that attempt to explain or predict certain behaviors or actions. Most of the earlier studies concentrated on bankruptcy explanations and predictions. Only since the 1960s have researchers attempted to analyze mergers by using accounting information, particularly financial ratios. Most of these studies do not focus on a particular industry, but on all bankruptcies or mergers over a specific period of time.

Presented here is a summary of previous studies. First, the use of accounting data for model building and predictions is discussed. Then, we explain how discriminant analysis evolved. Finally, the adaptation of this type of research to a particular industry—in this case the health care industry—is explained.

Probably the earliest study employing accounting numbers in an attempt to make decisions regarding the status of firms was published by Rosendale in 1908. His concern was the extension of bank loans to companies and their ability to repay these loans. His work included such financial statement analyses as rates of gross profit, bad debts, dividends, and the ratio of quick assets to liabilities.[1] For use in his analysis, he devised standard forms that resembled, in substance, the balance sheet of today, with particular emphasis on liquidity or quick assets.

Fitzpatrick may have been the first to employ numerous accounting ratios to compare successful firms and unsuccessful firms. He compared the ratios of 19 successful companies with 19 failed companies in the same industries over the period from 1919 to 1928.[2] Ratios that he employed included:

- current ratio
- quick ratio
- sales to fixed assets
- sales to inventories
- sales to receivables
- sales to net worth
- net worth to debt
- net worth to fixed assets
- inventories to receivables
- net profit to net worth
- current assets to total assets
- fixed assets to total assets
- other assets to total assets

Obviously, this is a rather lengthy list of ratios and appears to be the first attempt to discriminate between firms. But, also, it can be seen that most of the ratios involve analysis of only the balance sheet structure of the firms. Industries that were studied included meat-packing, confection, cereal, piano manufacturing, writing paper manufacturing, cane sugar and bananas, agricultural implement manufacturers, footwear, and others. Fitzpatrick concluded that in every industry the successful firms' ratios were significantly better than the unsuccessful firms' ratios. *He also concluded that ratios such as net worth to debt and net profit to net worth were very significant.*[3] A bothersome problem encountered by Fitzpatrick was that not every company published financial statements, particularly the failed companies.

A study by Smith and Winakor in 1935 of the financial structure of unsuccessful companies emphasized the current position of firms as well as composition of assets, liabilities, and net worth and also analyzed revenue. The study involved 183 companies that failed between 1923 and 1931. Fifteen percent of these companies were in manufacturing. Once again, many companies did not publish financial statements, particularly their income statements, or, if published, the statements were incomplete. Ratios employed included:

- the current ratio
- cash to total assets
- asset composition ratios
- liability and net worth composition ratios
- net earnings to total assets
- net income to net worth
- sales to total assets
- dividend policies
- working capital to total assets
- current asset liquidity
- current liabilities to total assets

Smith and Winaker found that the ratios working capital to total assets, cash to total assets, current asset liquidity, and current liabilities to total assets were found to be the best indicators of imminent failure for unsuccessful companies as they approached bankruptcy.[4] Merwin did a similar study of firms in five different industries over the period 1926 to 1932. He compared the mean ratios of continuing firms with those of discontinued firms and the difference in the means as much as six years before discontinuance. These differences increased as the year of the discontinuance approached.[5] Probably the first study to analyze financial ratios not just to explain failure but to predict failure was by Beaver in 1966.[6] As Beaver stated, his concern was that financial ratios can be predictors of significant events—not only bankruptcy. As stated by Ijiri and Jaedicke, the primary purpose of accounting data is to assist the reader in making rational financial decisions. Therefore, accounting information should be objective and realizable.[7] In Beaver's study, 30 ratios were analyzed comparing failed and non-failed firms. Ratios used included:

- *cash-flow ratios* (such as cash flow to assets and cash flow to sales);
- *net-income ratios* (such as net income to sales and net income to net worth);
- *debt to total-asset ratios* (such as current liabilities to total assets and total liabilities to total assets);

- *liquid-asset to total-asset ratios* (such as cash to total assets and current assets to total assets);
- *liquid-asset to current debt ratios* (such as cash to current liabilities and quick assets to current liabilities); and
- *turnover ratios* (such as cash to sales and total assets to sales).[8]

As can be seen, many of these ratios were studied by researchers early in the 1900s. The factors found to have the most significance were cash flow to total debt, net income to total assets, total debt to total assets, working capital to total assets, current ratio, and no-credit intervals. *The ratio with the best ability to predict was found to be cash-flow to total-debt.* Beaver's conclusion was that ratio analysis can be useful for at least five years before failure, but not all ratios have the same degree of success in predicting failure.[9]

In a later paper, Beaver, Kennelly, and Voss related prediction ability to what is generally regarded as the purpose of accounting data—the facilitation of decision making.[10] They defined predictive power as "the ability to generate operational implications (i.e., predictions) and to have those predictions subsequently verified by empirical evidence."[11]

USE OF ACCOUNTING NUMBERS
TO PREDICT TAKEOVERS

Since the late 1960s, the accounting literature has extended the use of accounting information from predicting bankruptcy to the prediction and analysis of mergers and acquisitions. The earlier papers laid the foundation of the use of financial data and ratios and their relevance to the decision-making process, although those papers and more recent papers note the limitations of this data.

One of the first papers to analyze takeover probability was written by Vance in 1969. The factors Vance advanced as those that would make a company an attractive takeover target included a low price-earnings ratio, high liquidity, excess debt capacity, and stability of earnings.[12] He calculated "danger zones" for companies for these ratios and found that 17 of 21 companies that were extended tender offers fell into this zone. Other nonfinancial factors found to be important were a dominant market position in an attractive growth sector of the economy and a company's unknowingly presenting a key piece of data to another's planned integration program.[13]

Gort studied mergers over the period 1951 to 1959, restricting his study to manufacturing firms. His findings were that economic disturbances (discrepancies in valuation for income-producing assets arising from differences in expectations about future income streams and the risks associated with expected income) generate discrepancies in value of the type needed to produce mergers. He concluded that these conditions appear much more frequently in periods of high security prices than those of low security prices. Variances in security prices were found to be the most important economic shock that increases the dispersion of values and thus leads to more mergers.[14]

Taussig and Hayes studied 50 companies that had been tendered takeover offers over the period July 1, 1956 to January 1, 1967 and paired them with another 50 companies of similar sales size in an attempt to discover whether accounting policies characterized companies that were susceptible to takeover bids. The results of their study were that firms subjected to takeover bids over the period analyzed had no significant differences in relative sizes of inventories, the ratio of net fixed assets to total assets, and the relationship between book ratio and market value of a company's stock, as compared to the control companies. They concluded that assets of firms subjected to takeover bids were valued on a similar basis (or not significantly different from) similarly sized firms in their industry. But they *did find* that companies vulnerable to take-over bids *had excess* liquid assets and a *correspondingly high quick ratio* and had a lower return on net worth.[15]

Lewellyn in 1971 focused on the potential opportunity for corporate growth as a reason for firms to merge. Some of the opportunities that firms may take advantage of would include economies to scale, implementing a more complete product line, complementary research or technological expertise, and greater administrative efficiency.[16] Also, by merging, firms would be able to decrease earnings variability of the combined company as long as the combining enterprises did not have earnings streams that were perfectly correlated. Finally, firms would be able to coinsure each other's debt and therefore decrease the profitability of default.[17]

Mueller was one of the first researchers to study mergers and offer as a reason for mergers the synergistic effects of the consolidation. Mueller felt that by "risk-pooling," overall risk of the merged firms would be greatly decreased. Similar to what Lewellyn said, Mueller offered that the risks surrounding the earnings streams of the two merging companies would be reduced when the earnings streams were combined. Also, pooling has the effect of offering to the stockholders a more diversified portfolio. Other synergistic benefits cited by Mueller include the combination of the management of the two firms into one and greater financial opportunities available to the merged firms because of larger annual cash flow and increased access to outside funds.[18]

Two studies attempted to determine why companies would pay a premium for another firm. These studies attempted to support the opponents of Lewellyn and Mueller because the two studies analyze the effects of synergy in two merger transactions. Nielsen and Melicher studied the possible merger synergy motives underlying the payment of merger premiums when they sampled 128 large industrial mergers between 1960 and 1969. The variables they found to be significant to differentiate between large and small overpayments were the percentage change in earnings per share, the size-adjusted change in cash flow rate, the acquiring firm's premerger, cash flow rate, and the acquiring firm's premerger operating profit rate.[19] They also concluded that the higher the variability in earnings, the higher the premiums paid for the acquired firm.[20]

In a later paper, Melicher and Neilsen cited anticipated benefits of acquiring firms for entering into specific mergers and found that the most often cited reasons were extensions of existing product lines, anticipation of operating economies with financial benefits following marketing benefits.[21]

In the late 1970s and into the 1980s, researchers continued to analyze mergers in an attempt to identify those factors that made a firm a takeover target. Merjos analyzed 70 takeover attempts made in 1977-1978. She found that common characteristics of the target companies to include a strong current position measured by current ratio, but generally cash was below average for these same companies. Also, debt burdens were no worse than average, profitability seemed to be above average with earnings growing in recent years before the bids, return on equity was seen to be above average, and diversification was a major motive of the tender bids.[22]

Shrieves and Stevens sampled mergers during the period from 1948 to 1971 found the following factors to be significant in choosing target firms:

- working capital/total assets
- retained earnings/total assets
- earnings before interest and tax/total assets
- market value of equity/book value of total debt
- sales/total assets[23]

Palepu sampled the period 1971 to 1979 using logit analysis to predict takeover targets. Variables employed in his model included:

- average excess return
- return on equity
- growth
- liquidity
- leverage
- size
- market-to-market book ratio
- price earnings ratio

He concluded that the variables' average excess return, growth, and size were statistically significant, indicating that inefficiency and smaller size would lead to an increase in a firm's probability of being acquired.[24]

Lin concluded that variables such as lower growth and leverage, higher liquidity, smaller size, high dividend payment ratio, low operating loss carry forward, similar activity ratios, and under valuation of assets increase a firm's probability of being acquired.[25]

USE OF DISCRIMINANT ANALYSIS TO PREDICT TAKEOVER TARGETS

Multiple discriminant analysis "involves the linear coordination of the two (or more) independent variables that will discriminate best between the *a priori* defined groups. This is achieved by the statistical decision rule of maximizing the between-group variance relative to the within-group variance, this relationship is expressed as the ratio of between-group to within-group variance."[26] The objectives of discriminant analysis include deriving a score that will separate two or more groups using independent variables.

Discriminant analysis, therefore, can be considered either a type of profile analysis or an analytical predictive technique. In either case, the technique is most appropriate when there is a simple categorical dependent variable and several metrically scaled independent variables.[27]

This technique has been adapted since the 1970s in the accounting literature to differentiate between possible takeover targets and those that are not targets. The first use of discriminant analysis found in the literature was probably by R. A. Fisher in 1936.[28] Others followed, with the most common usage of discriminant analysis being to predict bankruptcy by attempting to differentiate bankrupt firms and nonbankrupt firms by analyzing financial ratios.

Not until the 1970s was discriminant analysis used for other purposes, such as for separating takeover targets from nontakeover targets. Following is a summary of some of the research that emphasizes discriminant analysis followed by a summary of the research done on mergers and acquisitions.

One of the first papers published on using discriminant analysis for predictions was the landmark paper by Altman in 1968. He attempted to assess the quality of ratio analysis as an analytical tool. He also attempted to predict corporate bankruptcy by investigating a set of financial and economic ratios limited to manufacturing corporations.[29] The new quality offered by Altman was to not only isolate those ratios that portend financial difficulty and possible bankruptcy but also to attach weights to their relative importance. The sample selected by Altman was composed of 66 corporations, 33 of which had declared bankruptcy. The period covered in the sample was 1946 to 1965. Nonbankrupt firms were selected on the basis of firm size in an attempt to match most closely the bankrupt group. The ratios were classified into the five standard groups of liquidity, profitability, leverage, solvency, and activity. His results were that five ratios did the best overall job in the prediction of corporate bankruptcy. The final discriminant function was:

X_1 = working capital/total assets
X_2 = retained earnings/total assets
X_3 = earnings before interest and taxes/total assets
X_4 = market value equity/book value of total debt
X_5 = sales/total assets
Z = overall index[30]

The results of this discriminant function were that the model correctly classified 79 percent of the sample firms as bankrupt or nonbankrupt. Altman concluded that based on his results "it is suggested that the bankruptcy prediction model is an accurate forecaster of failure up to two years prior to bankruptcy and that the accuracy diminished substantially as the lead time increases."[31]

After the Altman paper was published, the use of discriminant analysis in the accounting and finance literature grew tremendously and many authors employed this method in different areas. The use of multiple discriminant analysis in the merger and acquisition literature appeared in the early 1970s, shortly after the Altman study.

A paper by Simkowitz and Monroe in 1971 attempted to differentiate the financial profile of firms that were taken over to see if there was a method of providing a criterion for identifying firms with a high probability of being taken over.[32]

Their sample was composed of companies that were merged or bought and a second sample contained nonabsorbed firms. The period of study was between April 1, 1968 and December 31, 1968. Twenty-four firms were selected. An attempt to measure the firms' growth, size, profitability, leverage, dividend policy, and liquidity was made. The results of this study were that seven variables or ratios best offered discrimination between the observed groups. The variables were:

• market turnover of equity shares
• price-earnings ratios
• sales volume
• three-year average dividend payment
• three-year average annual percentage change in common equity

- dummy variable for negative earnings,
- three-year average common dividends/last year common equity[33]

This methodology resulted in 77 percent of the firms being correctly classified. *The variable found to be most important was the price-earnings ratio followed by the past three years' dividends.*

Singh studied takeovers that occurred during the period 1955 through 1960 for the electrical engineering, food, and nonelectrical engineering industries. The variables he used were:

- pre-tax profitability
- post-tax profitability
- dividend return
- productive return
- liquidity
- gearing
- retention ratio
- growth
- a valuation ratio

He found that the rates of return were the best discriminators between merged firms and nonmerged firms. The success rate of proper classification that Singh achieved approximated 65 percent. His classification success rate was significant at the 5 percent level for firms' short-term period and at the 10 percent level for long-term data.[34]

Stevens studied 80 firms during 1966, 40 of which were acquired and 40 of which were not acquired. He analyzed profitability, liquidity, activity, and leverage ratios and averaged them for the two reporting periods prior to the acquisition. A total of 20 accounting and financial ratios were employed in this study, similar to those used in previous studies. Samples were matched according to size and covered all industries.

After performing factor analysis and multiple discriminant analysis, Stevens was able to reduce the significant factors to four—earnings before interest and taxes/sale, net working capital/assets, sales/assets, and long-term liabilities/assets. The last ratio was found to be the most significant, meaning that acquired firms tended to have lower levels of leverage. This was the similar conclusion previously stated by Lewellyn.

The accuracy achieved by Stevens is this study was a total classification accuracy of 70 percent, which he found to be significant at the 0.001 level. He concluded that financial data can provide a measure to separate firms ripe for acquisition from those that are poor targets.[35]

Belkaoui studied Canadian firms during the period 1960 to 1968 in an attempt to identify the financial characteristics of companies that became takeover targets. He selected 25 companies, an amount that was restricted by the availability of the accounting data. He employed 17 ratios as potential predictors falling into the categories of nonliquid asset ratios, liquid assets to current debt, and liquid asset turnover. He chose these particular ratios based largely on their prior popularity in previous studies. *The ratios Belkaoui found to be the most significant or had the lowest error percentage results were net income/net worth and cash flow/net worth.* Discriminant analysis resulted in a predictive success rate of between 70 and 85 percent with the most significant variable being working capital/total assets.[36]

Wansley and Lane studied firms that merged during the period 1975 to 1977. A total of 83 mergers were analyzed using multiple discriminant analysis. Five variables were found to be significant:

- price-earnings ratio
- long-term debt to total assets
- natural log of net sales
- compound growth in net sales
- market value to book value

The authors concluded that acquired firms had smaller price-earnings ratios, used less debt, were smaller in size, were growing more rapidly, and had less market value in relation to book value than nonacquired firms. *The natural log of net sales was found to be the most significant variable followed by price-earnings ratio.* The success rate in proper classifications was approximately 69 percent. They concluded that firms with a high chance for acquisition may be successfully separated from companies with a low potential solely based on their financial characteristics.[37] Wansley followed with a study of 44 merged firms during the period 1975 and 1976. He employed 20 variable ratios in the areas of profitability, size, leverage, liquidity, price-earnings, stock market characteristics, market valuation, growth, activity, and dividend policy. Of these variables, five specific ratios were found to be most significant:

- price/earnings per share
- long-term debt/total assets
- natural log of net sales
- three-year compound growth in net sales
- market value per share/book value per share

But, Wansley did find that 17 of the 20 variables did seem to have some importance in differentiating high-potential firms from others. Accuracy of the model ranged approximately from 61 percent to 75 percent, depending on the model used.[38]

What appears to be the first analysis of merged firms using financial ratios by industry was performed by Omurtak in 1986. He studied 341 firms acquired over the period 1970 to 1983. These firms were classified into four industry groups: mining, manufacturing, trade, and services. He chose an initial set of 21 variables based on profitability, liquidity, leverage, activity, market valuation, stock market characteristics, size, and growth. A discriminant model was developed for each of these years prior to acquisition. The model found four variables to be most significant:

- common shares traded/common shares outstanding
- price per share-close/book value of assets per share
- long term liabilities/total assets
- natural log of net sales

The model was found to be statistically significant based on the F-test.[39] Next, Omurtak developed discriminant models within Standard Industrial Classification (SIC) codes. For the mining industry, the results of the discriminant analysis were not significant in discriminating between acquired firms and nonacquired firms. In the manufacturing industry, the discriminant analysis was effective in separating acquired firms from nonacquired firms. But in the trade industry and the service industry, the discriminant function was not effective.

Finally, Omurtak constructed industry-specific models using industry-specific variables. For the mining industry the variables were:

• market value/book value
• common shares traded/common shares outstanding
• growth in sales
• growth in net worth
• quick assets/current liabilities

These variables measured stock market characteristics, market valuation, growth, and liquidity. The predictive ability of this model was tested using 38 firms in a total group with half of the sample representing acquired firms and half representing nonacquired firms. The results of this function were that slightly less than 50 percent accuracy was achieved in correctly classifying between acquired firms and nonacquired firms one, two and three years prior to acquisition.

For the manufacturing industry, Omurtak used four variables:

• market value/book value
• common shares traded/common shares outstanding
• long-term liabilities/total assets
• natural log of net sales

The predictive power of the model was employed using 188 firms, half being acquired firms and half representing nonacquired. The accuracy of this model showed a 62 to 66 percent average in classifying correctly.

For the trade industry, Omurtak used the variables:

• market value/book value
• common shares trade/common shares outstanding
• a dummy variable for negative earnings
• growth in net worth
• natural log of net sales
• earnings before interest and taxes/total assets

Among the four industry groups studied, this group had the highest correct classification ratio, ranging from 58 percent correctly classified three years prior to merger and 73 percent one year prior to acquisition.

For the service industry the variables employed were:

- market value/book value
- market price/earnings per share
- quick assets/current liabilities
- sales/total assets

The classification accuracy of this model ranged from 65 percent to 70 percent. The most significant variables in the models were market activity and market valuation for the manufacturing industry, activity and growth in sales for the mining industry, dummy variables for negative earnings and market valuation for the trade industry, and liquidity and profitability in the service industry.

REFERENCE NOTES

1. William M. Rosendale, "Credit Department Methods," *The Bankers Magazine*, 1908, 186-187.

2. Paul J. Fitzpatrick, "A Comparison of the Ratios of Successful Industrial Enterprises with Those of Failed Companies," *The Certified Public Accountant*, October-December 1932, 598-605.

3. Ibid., October-December 1932, 731.

4. Raymond A. Smith and Arthur H. Winakor, *Changes in the Financial Structure of Unsuccessful Industrial Corporations*, University of Illinois: Bureau of Business Research, 1935, 7-40.

5. Charles Merwin, *Financing Small Corporations in Five Manufacturing Industries: 1926-32*, New York: Bureau of Economic Research, 1942, 25-40.

6. William F. Beaver, "Financial Ratios as Predictors of Failure," *Empirical Research in Accounting: Selected Studies, 1966*, University of Chicago: Institute of Professional Accounting, Graduate School of Business, 1967, 71-111.

7. Yuji Ijiri and Robert K. Jaedicke, "Reliability and Objectivity of Accounting Measurements," *The Accounting Review*, July 1966, 474-483.

8. Beaver, 78.

9. Ibid., 91.

10. William H. Beaver, John W. Kennelly, and William M. Voss, "Predictive Ability as a Criterion for the Evaluation of Accounting Data," *The Accounting Review*, October 1968, 67.

11. Ibid., 677.

12. Jack O. Vance, "Is Your Company a Take-over Target?" *Harvard Business Review*, May-June 1969, 94.

13. Ibid.

14. Michael Gort, "An Economic Disturbance Theory of Mergers," *Quarterly Journal of Economics*, November 1969, 626-628.

15. Russell A. Taussig and Samuel L. Hayes III, "Cash Take-Overs and Accounting Valuations," *The Accounting Review*, January 1968, 70-73.

16. Wilbur G. Lewellyn, "A Pure Financial Rationale for the Conglomerate Merger," *The Journal of Finance*, May 1971, 521.

17. Ibid., 523.

18. Dennis C. Mueller, "A Theory of Conglomerate Mergers," *Quarterly Journal of Economics*, November 1969, 643-653.

19. James F. Nielsen and Ronald W. Melicher, "A Financial Analysis of Acquisition and Merger Premiums," *Journal of Financial and Quantitative Analysis*, March 1973, 140-142.

20. Ibid., 143.

21. Ronald W. Melicher and James F. Neilsen, "Financial Factors That Affect Acquisition Prices," *Review of Business & Economic Research*, Winter 1977/8, 98.

22. Anna Merjos, "Takeover Targets," *Barrons*, May 15, 1978, 31-32.

23. Ronald E. Shrieves and Donald L. Stevens, "Bankruptcy Avoidance as a Motive for Merger," *Journal of Financial and Quantitative Analysis*, September 1979, 507.

24. Robert S. Harris, John F. Steward, David K. Guilky, and Willard T. Carleton, "Characteristics of Acquired Firms: Fixed and Random Coefficients Profit," *Southern Economic Journal*, July 1982, 177.

25. You-an Robert Lin, "The Use of Supplementing Accounting Disclosures for Corporate Takeover Targets Prediction" PhD diss. University of California, Los Angeles, 1989, 150-165.

26. Joseph F. Hair, Rolph E. Anderson, and Ronald L. Tatham, *Multivariate Data Analysis: With Readings*, New York: Macmillan Publishing Company, 1987, 75.

27. Ibid., 79.

28. R. A. Fisher, "The Use of Multiple Measurements in Taxonomic Problems," *Annals of Eugenics*, September 1936, 179-180.

29. Edward I. Altman, "Financial Ratios, Discriminant Analysis, and the Prediction of Corporate Bankruptcy," *The Journal of Finance*, September 1968, 589.

30. Ibid., 593-594.

31. Ibid., 604.

32. Michael Simkowitz and Robert J. Monroe, "A Discriminant Analysis Function for Conglomerate Targets," *The Southern Journal of Business*, November 1971, 16.

33. Ibid., 6-7.

34. Ajit Singh, *Takeovers: Their Relevance to the Stock Market and the Theory of the Firm*, Cambridge: Cambridge University Press, 1971, 114-119.

35. Donald L. Stevens, "Financial Characteristics of Merged Firms: A Multivariate Analysis," *Journal of Financial and Quantitative Analysis*, March 1973, 150-157.

36. Ahmed Belkaoui, "Financial Ratios as Predictors of Canadian Takeovers," *Journal of Business Finance & Accounting*, Spring 1978, 93-102.

37. James W. Wansley and William R. Lane, "A Financial Profile of Merged Firms," *Review of Business & Economic Research*, Fall 1984, 77-82.

38. James W. Wansley, "Discriminant Analysis and Merger Theory," *Review of Business & Economic Research*, Fall 1984, 77-82.

39. Sehra Saridereli Omurtak, "Financial Ratios as Predictors of Corporate Acquisition Candidates by Industry," PhD diss. University of Missouri, Rolla, 1986, 27-40.

40. Ibid., 54-64.

Chapter 3

Studies Performed on Hospitals

One of the earliest studies of merged hospitals was performed by Treat in 1973. He stated that "the current overriding problems in the delivery of health care are: (1) how to achieve effectiveness in terms of adequate quantity and quality of service; and (2) how to provide that service efficiently (i.e., at least cost)."[1] He quoted the National Commission of Community Health Services as saying as early as 1966 that "hospitals and allied facilities should explore every available additional means for improving management, increasing efficiency, and reducing cost. Such means should include systems of joint management and the exploration of the possibility of merging small hospitals."[2] Thus, the merging of hospitals was recommended in the 1960s, and research in this area has become prevalent. Treat attempted to compare hospital performance before and after a merger. He cited reasons for merger:

- to improve and expand the services offered by the hospital
- to ensure institutional survival
- to eliminate unnecessary duplication of facilities
- to improve utilization rates
- to modernize and expand facilities
- to enhance research programs
- to obtain economies of scale, synergy, and improved management[3]

Treat investigated the period 1956 to 1970. He compared the mean difference of 14 selected indicators of efficiency of merging and nonmerging hospitals. These measures included:

- *general factors* such as service available and patient admittance patterns

- *environmental factors* such as area medical facilities and demographics
- *physical facilities factors* such as age and condition of the plant
- *structural factors* such as size and managerial components
- *financing factors* such as utilization of capital and cost and revenue patterns
- *process factors* such as average length of stay and occupancy rate
- *education and research factors* such as numbers of interns and residents
- *outcome factors* such as cost per day and case and staff to patient ratio

Treat's findings were that *mergers tended to reduce efficiency while at the same time increasing effectiveness.* Inefficiencies were found in the areas of average cost per case, average cost per day, total expenses, and patient days, while favorable performance was found in the areas of bed quantities, services, and approvals.[4] Treat did not study the area of acquisition candidates and the analysis of accounting data to create a model to predict candidates but is one of the early, thorough analyses of merged hospitals and their performance.

In the early 1980s, several studies analyzed hospital performance in order to predict failure. One of the earliest papers was by Cleverly in 1981. He used financial ratio analysis in an attempt to predict financial failure when he studied a sample of New York State hospitals. He studied the standard financial ratios that fall into the categories of *liquidity* (current ratios, avid test ratio, collection period, average payment period), *capital structure* (long-term debt/fixed assets, long-term debt/equity, times interest earned, debt service coverage, cash flow to debt), *activity* (total asset turnover, fixed asset turnover, current asset turnover, inventory turnover), and *profitability* (mark-up, deductible, operating margin, nonoperating revenue contribution, return on assets).

A sample of failed hospitals was selected for the period 1973 to 1978. Many of the failed hospitals had to be eliminated from the study because of a lack of data, a problem confronted by most researchers when investigating hospitals. His objective was to determine whether or not financial ratios deteriorated one to four years prior to failure of hospitals and whether these ratios compared favorably or unfavorably to the industry averages. Of the 19 ratios examined, only four did not show decline between four years prior to failure and one year period to failure:

- long-term debt/fixed assets
- long-term debt/equity
- inventory turnover
- deductibles

Of the 19 variables only two were significant at the .10 level: average payment period and times interest earned. This was explained by the fact that most of the ratios had already deteriorated so badly by the year before failure that any further decline would be unlikely. The ratios may have predicted failure earlier than four years previous to the failure.[5]

Better results were found when Cleverly compared the industry average for these 19 variables with those of the hospitals that failed. He found six ratios that best discriminated failed hospitals versus industry averages:

- current ratios and test ratio
- average payment period
- operating margin
- return on assets
- times interest earned
- debt-service coverage[6]

Levitz and Brooke studied the financial ratios of independent versus system-affiliated hospitals in Iowa in 1981. They attempted to discover whether or not there were differences in the financial structure of these two groups of hospitals. They sampled 94 hospitals—74 independent and 20 affiliated.

They determined arithmetic means for 35 different ratios comprising the areas of liquidity, capital structure, financial activity, profitability, cost, and productivity. They included such variables as cost per day, cost per case, nurse pay per day, and admissions per bed. These arithmetic means were computed for the two groups and the t-test was used to determine significant differences between the two types of hospitals. The results of the study concluded that no significant differences between the two groups were observed for financial performance measures, but that a higher level of debt coverage was noted on the part of system-owned hospitals. In fact, the only significant differences found between contract-managed and system-owned hospitals were for the salary expense per patient day and salary expense per admission, both being higher for system-affiliated hospitals.

When comparing freestanding hospitals with system-affiliated hospitals more differences were noted. All measures of capital structure (equity financing, long-term debt/equity, long-term debt/fixed assets, cash flow/total liabilities) were significantly different between the two groups. Other significant differences included mean values on rate of return and measures of profitability, and total costs per case, which favored freestanding hospitals.[7]

These studies (Cleverly and Levitz and Brooke) were early attempts to study and analyze financial ratios for hospitals. As has been shown above, the accounting and finance literature has abundant analyses of financial ratios for all industries, but not many industry-specific analyses. Some papers attempted to analyze merged hospitals employing financial ratio analysis and to rectify this problem.

Mullner and Anderson studied merged hospitals from 1980 to 1985 in an attempt to describe the environmental characteristics of hospitals that combined and to examine whether the overall financial position of the hospitals changed. Financial ratio analysis was performed before and after the merger. The ratios employed were confined to the current ratio, the total margin ratio, and the net-to-gross-patient-revenue ratio. A total of 55 acquired hospitals and 45 acquiring hospitals were studied. The authors found that 91 percent of acquiring hospitals and 71 percent of acquired hospitals were community hospitals. Also, the largest percentage of acquired hospitals were of the smallest bed size. Other environmental factors studied by Mullner and Anderson included ownership type, location, metropolitan versus non metropolitan, and community size of the hospital area. The authors found that hospitals involved in mergers or consolidations had ratios that were close to industry averages both before and after the merger and that the effect of the mergers was small.[8] They concluded that, "no clear financial gains or losses characterized merging or consolidating hospitals either before or after merger or consolidation."[9] Of course, they limited their study severely by studying only these financial ratios and they did not attempt to find any consistency in the ratios to determine whether a specific type of hospital would be a possible target.

One study attempted to determine how prices are set in hospital acquisitions. McCue, McCue, and Wheeler studied 37 mergers that took place over the period 1978 to 1984 primarily in the south and southwest regions of the United States. The variables used included:

- cash flow per bed
- age of facility
- occupancy rate
- county income
- a competition measure
- a variable that measures a possible shift in market value over time

They applied ordinary least squares regression models to determine means and standard deviations of the variables. Their results indicated that market price paid per bed was significantly positively related to county income and occupancy rate and negatively to age of plant. The R^2 showed that approximately 35 percent of the variation in market price per bed was explained by the variables cash flow per bed, age of plant, county income, occupancy rate, competition, and reduction by date. A second regression was run to explain premiums paid per bed and it was found that only age of the facility significantly affected premium paid above book value per bed. The cash flow of the facility, the level of competition, county income, occupancy rate, and the prospective payment had no impact on the prices paid per bed.[10]

SUMMARY OF CHAPTERS 2 AND 3

The use of financial ratios in analyzing a company's performance has been in the accounting and finance literature since early in the twentieth century. At that time, it was used to make credit decisions for individuals by banks and other lending institutions. Then the use of financial ratios was extended to predict failure or nonfailure of firms. In this regard, Beaver's study is the most quoted study for setting the foundation for future research in this area.

Altman then followed with an often-quoted paper in the literature by emphasizing discriminant function to failed and nonfailed firms and derived a Z-score and equation. Other researchers extended these two works greatly over the following 20 to 25 years. Discriminant analysis has become very popular in the literature when attempting to show differences between two groups or samples. The use of discriminant analysis has been extended in analysis of mergers and merger candidates.

Studies have been presented that show the results of their attempts to identify takeover targets. These studies have generally been performed across industries and few have focused on a particular one or few industries.

Finally, hospitals have been analyzed in the literature starting in the 1970s. These studies have attempted to analyze successful versus unsuccessful hospitals as well as the financial profile of hospitals before merger or acquisition and the financial profile after acquisitions. The financial analysis performed has frequently been below that done by researchers who analyze mergers and acquisitions across industries. This book attempts to analyze hospitals that have been acquired in the state of California over the period 1980 to 1992. Statistical analysis has been performed in the financial data in an attempt to discriminate those hospitals that were targeted for takeover with a sample of like-sized hospitals that were not targeted for takeover during the same period of time. The analysis will be much more vigorous than that which was performed on hospitals in the studies summarized above. The goal is to discover whether there are common financial positions or conditions for acquired hospitals and to create a model that can be employed for future possible targeted hospitals.

The health care industry is the second most active in terms of mergers and acquisitions. Because of this high level of activity, there is a need for an accurate predictive model. Previous studies have shown inconsistent results. This study attempts to develop a more accurate model.

REFERENCE NOTES

1. Thomas Frank Treat, "A Study of the Characteristics and Performance of Merged Hospitals in the United States," PhD diss. Texas A&M University, December 1973, 3.

2. Ibid., 8-9.

3. Ibid., 147-152.

4. Ibid., 192-259.

5. William O. Cleverly, "Financial Ratios: Summary Indicators for Management Decision Making," *Hospital & Health Services Administration*, Special 1, 1981, 27-44.

6. Ibid., 46.

7. Gary S. Levitz and Paul P. Brooke Jr., "Independent versus System-Affiliated Hospitals: A Comparative Analysis of Financial Performance, Cost, and Productivity," *Health Services Research*, August 1985, 318-334.

8. Ross M. Mullner and Ronald M. Anderson, "A Descriptive and Financial Ratio Analysis of Merged and Consolidated Hospitals: United States 1980-1985," in *Advances in Health Economics and Health Services Research*, edited by Richard M. Scheffler and Louis F. Rossiter, Greenwich, CT: Jai Press, 1987, 43-56.

9. Ibid., 58.

10. Michael J. McCue, Tom McCue, and John R. C. Wheeler, "An Assessment of Hospital Acquisition Prices," *Inquiry*, Summer 1988, 291-294.

Chapter 4

Data Collection and Analysis

SOURCE DOCUMENTS

The data analyzed in this study were obtained from annual hospital reporting of financial information to the Office of Statewide Health Planning and Development (OSHPD) in Sacramento, California. As stated in their publication:

> . . . all non-federal hospitals licensed in California are required by Part 1.8 of the Health and Safety code to establish and use the hospital uniform accounting system prescribed by the Office. Annual financial statements and utilization reports are then submitted by these hospitals to the Office within four months of the close of their fiscal years.[1]

The data collected by OSHPD is then made available to the public in annual publications. The data is published in three annual volumes that assess different geographic areas. Volume 1 covers the areas of Northern California, Golden Empire, North Bay, West Bay, East Bay, North San Joaquin, Santa Clara County, and Mid Coast. Volume 2 covers the Los Angeles County area and Volume 3 includes Central California, Ventura, Santa Barbara, Inland Counties, Orange County and San Diego/Imperial areas. The reporting periods covered by these publications usually run from June to the following June. Data were collected in this study by utilizing all three annual publications of the Office during the fiscal years from 1979/80 through 1990/91. Since there is usually more than a one-year delay in the publication of these books and date of the financial statements, the last period available for analysis for this study was the 1990/91 fiscal year.

Information available in these publications include summarized balance sheets and income statements as well as some financial ratios. For the balance sheet, titles such as short term assets, net property, plant and equipment, construction in progress, other assets, short-term liabilities, long-term liabilities, and equity are given each year with amounts. For the income statement, totals are given for gross patient revenue, deductions from revenue, other operating revenue, total operating expenses, net income from operations, nonoperating revenue and expenses, income taxes, extraordinary items, and net income. Financial ratios calculated include the current ratio, acid test ratio, days in accounts receivable, bad debt rate, long-term debt/total assets, debt service coverage, fixed asset growth rate, net return on operating assets, operating margin, turnover of operating assets and net property, plant, and equipment per bed.

Additional ratios were computed for this study using the balance sheet and income statement data and are presented below.

Lists of hospitals that have consolidated with parent and subsidiary identified are also published by OSHPD. These lists were instrumental in identifying those hospitals to be analyzed in this work. A total of 29 purchased hospitals for which separate financial data were available were identified over the period 1980-1992. Many of the consolidations and purchases were of Kaiser Foundation Hospitals where full financial information was not available. The list of purchased hospitals and their parents in this study appear in Table 4.1.

These were the only hospitals with sufficient financial information available, particularly for the subsidiaries, on which valid tests could be performed.

EMPIRICAL DATA

For all the parents and subsidiaries, information was accumulated for up to five years before the merger date. Ratios were calculated in this study during the five year period up to the merger. Ratios published by the OSHPD as well as ratios computed from the published financial data are presented. Ratios published by OSHPD included:

- current ratio
- acid test ratio
- days in accounts receivable
- bad debt rate
- long-term debt/total assets
- debt service coverage
- fixed asset growth
- return on assets
- operating margin
- asset turnover
- property plant and equipment/bed
- length of patient stays, and
- occupancy rate

Ratios calculated for this study included:

- natural log of total revenue
- net income/equity
- total revenue/total assets
- long-term debt/equity
- short-term debt/total assets, and
- net working capital/total assets.

These ratios were similar to those employed by the researchers in the literature survey (Chapters 2 and 3). Simkowitz and Monroe,[2] Stevens,[3] and Wansley and Lane[4] all used similar ratios in their analyses. Discriminant analysis was utilized in all these studies and was the major statistical analysis employed in this study. Data for the above-listed takeover targets were accumulated as well as data for hospitals that were not taken over.

The method used to select hospitals that were not taken over was to find hospitals of similar annual revenue. To be comparable, revenue needed to be very similar in the year prior to takeover. Data were collected for these firms for up to the same five years prior to takeover as for the hospitals. Also, hospitals in the same geographic area were chosen when possible. Data was calculated from the same source: the Office of Statewide Health Planning and Development *Annual Reports of Hospitals*. The same types of ratios were calculated for the nontargeted hospitals as had been collected for the

TABLE 4.1. Purchased Hospitals with Separate Financial Data, by Date of Acquisition

Date	Purchased Hospital	Parent
1982	1. Sierra Care Center	Sonora Community Hospital
7/31/84	2. Santa Rosa General Hospital	Santa Rosa Memorial Hospital
9/17/84	3. Doctor's Hospital of Lakewood-Clark Avenue	Doctor's Hospital of Lakewood-South Street
9/30/84	4. Memorial Hospital, Ceres	Memorial Hospital, Modesto
1/01/85	5. Beverly Glen Hospital	Beverly Hills Medical Center
1/23/85	6. The Garden Campus	California Pacific Medical Center
7/01/85	7. O'Connor Hospital at Campbell	O'Connor Hospital
1/07/86	8. Crystal Springs Rehabilitation Center	San Mateo General Hospital
4/08/86	9. Pinecrest Hospital	Santa Barbara Cottage Hospital
11/01/86	10. Riverside Community Hospital Knollwood Center	Riverside Community Hospital
1/01/87	11. Community Hospital Recovery Center	Community Hospital of the Monterey Peninsula
2/01/87	12. Modesto City Hospital	Doctor's Medical Center
2/16/87	13. Simi Valley Community Hospital	Simi Valley Adventist Hospital
8/07/88	14. Ukiah General Hospital	Ukiah Adventist Hospital
1/01/89	15. Marshall Hale Hospital	Children's Hospital of San Francisco
1/27/89	16. Hollywood Presbyterian Hospital	Queen of Angels Medical Center
7/31/89	17. French Hospital Medical Center	Kaiser Foundation, San Francisco
9/01/89	18. Peralta Hospital	Samuel Merritt Hospital
10/31/89	19. Rancho Encino Hospital	Ami Tarzana Regional Medical Center
12/31/89	20. Herrick Hospital Health Center	Alta Bates Hospital
3/08/90	21. Dominican Community Hospital of Santa Cruz	Dominican Santa Cruz Hospital
4/26/90	22. Mission Oakes Hospital	Good Samaritan of Santa Clara

5/31/90	23. Ontario Community Hospital	Doctors' Hospital of Montclair
6/19/90	24. Doctors' Hospital of Santa Ana	Santa Ana Hospital
9/15/90	25. Lodi Memorial Hospital-West	Lodi Memorial Hospital
9/01/91	26. Mission Hospital	Community Hospital Huntington Park
9/12/91	27. Alvarado Parkway Institute	Alvarado Community Hospital
12/31/91	28. Van Nuys Community Hospital	Hollywood Community Hospital
2/29/92	29. Providence Hospital	Merritt Hospital

Note: Postmerger names are used because data are represented in this manner by the OSHPD.

targeted hospitals. The accounting numbers were then entered into the NCSS statistical package.[5]

Discriminant analysis on the data was performed for the periods one year before the merger to five years before merger in an attempt to differentiate one group from the other. All the mergers occurred and the data were collected during the period 1981 to 1991. Data for the period prior to 1981 are not published in the same information format as later years in the annual publication of OSHPD.

Therefore, accounting ratios were not able to be computed for periods preceding 1981. Since most of the takeovers occurred from the mid-1980s on, the lack of a full five years of information was not a factor in more than one or two cases. The hospitals chosen to compare to those taken over are listed in Table 4.2.

ANALYSIS OF RESULTS

As stated above, data were entered into a discriminant analysis program in an attempt to differentiate merged (target) firms from firms not purchased. An equal number of merged and nonmerged hospitals over the previous ten years were entered into the program. Nonmerged hospitals were chosen on the basis of similar geographic area and similar size according to revenue.

TABLE 4.2. Takeover Target Hospitals and Correlative Nontakeover Hospitals

Takeover	No Takeover
1. Van Nuys Community Hospital	Newhall Community Hospital
2. Santa Rosa General Hospital	Alisal Community Hospital
3. Hollywood Presbyterian Hospital	Certinela Hospital Medical Center
4. Providence Hospital	Dameron Hospital
5. Beverly Glen Hospital	Crossroads Hospital
6. Ukiah General Hospital	Sutter Coast Hospital
7. The Garden Campus	Los Banos Community Hospital
8. Marshall Hale Hospital	Petaluma Valley Hospital
9. French Hospital Medical Center	Alameda Hospital
10. Crystal Springs Rehabilitation Center	George L. Mee Memorial Hospital
11. Herrick Hospital Health Center	Los Medanos Community Hospital
12. Peralta Hospital	Fairmont Hospital
13. Lodi Memorial Hospital-West	Amador Hospital
14. Memorial Hospital, Ceres	Novato Community Hospital
15. Modesto City Hospital	Merced Community Medical Center
16. Sierra Care Center	Mark Twain Hospital
17. O'Connor Hospital at Campbell	St. Joseph's Oak Park Hospital
18. Mission Oakes Hospital	Wheeler Hospital
19. Dominican Community Hospital of Santa Cruz	Arroyo Grande Community Hospital
20. Community Hospital Recovery Center	Community Hospital of Salinas
21. Pinecrest Hospital	Shicks Shadel Hospital
22. Simi Valley Community Hospital	Ojai Valley Community Hospital
23. Rancho Encino Hospital	Burbank Community Hospital
24. Mission Hospital	College Hospital
25. Doctor's Hospital of Lakewood-Clark Avenue	Community Hospital of Gardenia
26. Riverside Community Hospital Knollwood Center	Fullerton Community Hospital
27. Ontario Community Hospital	Inland Valley Regional Medical Center
28. Doctor's Hospital of Santa Ana	Anaheim General Hospital
29. Alvarado Parkway Institute	Coronado Hospital

This analysis covered the periods of one year, two years, three years, four years, and five years prior to the takeover.

SIGNIFICANT VARIABLES PRIOR TO MERGER

One Year Prior to Merger

As shown in Table 4.3 for the period one year prior to merger, the variables that were found to be significant were current ratio, bad debt rate (as a percentage of gross patient revenue), long-term debt/total assets, return on assets, operating margin, net income/equity, and short-term debt/total assets.

According to Table 4.3, the factor with the largest weight was current ratio (30.39508). The other positive factors dealt with long-term debt/total assets, return on assets, and short-term debt/total

TABLE 4.3. Significant Variables One Year Prior to Merger

Factor	Weights		F-Value
	Merged	Nonmerged	
Current Ratio	30.39508	21.58451	9.9
Bad Debt Rate	— 1.020957	— 0.3263474	6.5
Long-Term Debt/ Total Assets	0.4631253	2.996372	12.6
Return on Assets	3.872039	2.408948	38.0
Operating Margin	— 5.493266	— 3.415032	30.1
Net Income/Equity	— 0.6900123	— 0.3567182	29.4
Short-Term Debt/ Total Assets	1.910542	1.264753	24.0

assets. These results are supported by the findings of other research-ers (e.g., Taussig and Hayes, 1968; Merjos, 1978; Stevens, 1973) in that targeted firms often had strong current ratios and were more heavily in debt than nontargeted firms. Negative weights were attached to the factors bad debt rate, operating margin, and net income/equity. This supports the conclusion of others (e.g., Vance, 1969; Belkaoui, 1978; Wansley and Lane, 1984) that targeted firms are often losing money at the time of the takeover.

The success rate of properly classifying firms as merged or non-merged was significant the year before merger. Table 4.4 summa-rizes this success rate.

The overall Wilk's lambda for this function was 0.1338. Wilk's lambda is equal to $1-R^2$. It varies from one to zero. Values near one imply low predictability, while values close to zero imply high predictability.[6]

Two Years Prior to Merger

Results of the discriminant analysis for two years prior to merger are as follows. The same variables were employed in the analysis: current ratio, bad debt rate, long-term debt/total assets, return on assets, operating margin, net income/equity, and short-term debt/to-tal assets. The weights and F-values for two years prior to merger are shown in Table 4.5.

From these results, none of the variables found to be significant one year prior to merger were found to be significant two years prior to merger. Both the weights and the F-values are not signifi-cant. The only factor that has a significant F-value in the discrimi-nant function was the natural log of sales (F-value of 4.6). Even with the low significance of the seven variables, the classification of merged versus nonmerged was still relatively good. In this case the success rate is summarized in Table 4.6. The overall Wilk's lambda increased to 0.6565 during the second year before merger.

Three Years Prior to Merger

The same seven variables were employed by the discriminant program for the period three years prior to merger. Table 4.7 sum-

TABLE 4.4. Predictive Success Rate One Year Before Merger

Factor	Merged	Nonmerged
Predicted to Merge	16	2
Predicted Not to Merge	2	27
TOTAL	18	29
Success Rate	89%	93%

TABLE 4.5. Significant Variables Two Years Prior to Merger

Factor	Weights		F-Value
	Merged	Nonmerged	
Current Ratio	1.981174	2.364078	0.4
Bad Debt Rate	0.077044	.225137	1.7
Long-Term Debt/ Total Assets	0.45725	0.025464	0.6
Return on Assets	.4013201	0.2909721	0.9
Operating Margin	−.5346213	−.3658217	0.7
Net Income/Equity	−0.001595	0.016351	0.6
Short-Term Debt/ Total Assets	0.077416	0.071684	0.1

marizes the statistical results obtained. As in the case for two years prior to merger, for three years prior to merger none of the variables are considered significant. The only variable that proved to be significant is fixed asset growth (F-value of 5.7)[7] The Wilk's lambda three years prior to merger has increased to 0.6721.

The success rate of properly classifying merged versus nonmerged firms three years prior to merger using the original seven variables are summarized in Table 4.8.

TABLE 4.6. Predictive Success Rate Two Years Before Merger

Factor	Merged	Nonmerged
Predicted to Merge	16	4
Predicted Not to Merge	2	26
TOTAL	18	30
Success Rate	89%	87%

TABLE 4.7. Significant Variables Three Years Prior to Merger

	Weights		
Factor	Merged	Nonmerged	F-Value
Current Ratio	2.043135	2.676359	2.5
Bad Debt Rate	.4745748	.6894092	2.7
Long-Term Debt/ Total Assets	0.092672	0.069227	0.7
Return on Assets	.2145794	.2848477	0.4
Operating Margin	−.2994441	−.2649512	0.0
Net Income/Equity	−0.000559	−0.007397	1.6
Short-Term Debt/ Total Assets	0.062560	0.075374	1.0

Even though the factors were not considered to be significant in the discriminant function, the success rate of predicting whether a merger would take place or not is still relatively good (68 percent and 77 percent).

Four Years Prior to Merger

Results of the test for four years prior to merger testing the same variables and hospitals as were used for one year prior to merger in Table 4.9.

TABLE 4.8. Predictive Success Rate Three Years Before Merger

Factor	Merged	Nonmerged
Predicted to Merge	13	6
Predicted Not to Merge	6	20
TOTAL	19	26
Success Rate	68%	77%

TABLE 4.9. Significant Variables Four Years Prior to Merger

	Weights		
Factor	Merged	Nonmerged	F-Value
Current Ratio	1.357363	1.125289	0.8
Bad Debt Rate	.3213706	.2963162	0.1
Long-Term Debt/ Total Assets	0.094547	0.084688	0.2
Return on Assets	.1466019	.1623168	0.1
Operating Margin	−.1434003	−0.038856	1.0
Net Income/Equity	−0.007688	−0.012877	0.4
Short-Term Debt/ Total Assets	.0897661	0.098917	0.3

The trend of the factors becoming less significant has been repeated in these results. All seven variables have become insignificant again and the only factor of significance four years prior to merger was days in accounts receivable (F-value of 4.3). The Wilk's lambda has increased further to 0.7992.

Although the factors became less significant in the model, the predictive rate according to proper classification as merged or nonmerged continues to be relatively good—as Table 4.10 suggests. The accuracy has decreased quite a bit from the previous years.

Five Years Prior to Merger

Finally, the same tests were performed on the data for five years prior to merger. The same seven variables were employed in the model. Results appear in Table 4.11.

Once again, all the factors that were significant in the original functions one year prior to merger are insignificant five years prior to merger. In fact, none of the factors employed proved to be significant in this scenario. The overall Wilk's lambda has increased again, this time to 0.8513.

TABLE 4.10. Predictive Success Rate Four Years Before Merger

Factor	Merged	Nonmerged
Predicted to Merge	12	10
Predicted Not to Merge	10	17
TOTAL	22	27
Success Rate	55%	63%

TABLE 4.11. Significant Variables Five Years Prior to Merger

	Weights		
Factor	Merged	Nonmerged	F-Value
Current Ratio	6.785572	6.438477	0.4
Bad Debt Rate	.6820685	.6633766	0.0
Long-Term Debt/ Total Assets	.1996382	.1793405	0.8
Return on Assets	.2960492	.2796331	0.0
Operating Margin	−.3849141	−.3283038	0.2
Net Income/Equity	−0.013707	−0.008446	0.4
Short-Term Debt/ Total Assets	.4984985	.5134127	0.1

The success rate of classifying merged versus nonmerged hospitals five years prior to merger can be summarized in Table 4.12.

Therefore, for the periods four years prior to merger and five years prior to merger, the success rate of properly classifying hospitals as merged or nonmerged is not much above 50 percent as was the case in the other three years.

Also, for the period one year after merger, t-tests were performed to determine which variables were materially different from the point of view of the buyer or parent. The results of this test appear in Table 4.13.

Thus, the variables that were significantly different for the parent one year before and one year after the merger proved to be:

- current ratio (changing from 3.33 to 2.61)
- acid test ratio (decreasing from an average of 1.62 to an average of .90)
- debt service coverage ratio (increasing from an average of 9.07 to an average of 121.01)
- fixed asset growth (growing from an average of 19.03 to an average of 32.16)
- net income/equity (decreasing from an average of 13.51 percent to a negative .70 percent)
- net income/total assets (decreasing from 170.74 to 135.23), and
- long-term debt/equity (increasing from an average of 107.89 to 168.83).

TABLE 4.12. Predictive Success Rate Five Years Before Merger

Factor	Merged	Nonmerged
Predicted to Merge	12	10
Predicted Not to Merge	8	15
TOTAL	20	25
Success Rate	60%	60%

TABLE 4.13. T-Test Results One Year After Merger

Variable	T-value	F-value
Current Ratio	0.93	6.819401
Acid Test Ratio	1.01	15.75881
Days in Accounts Receivable	−1.21	1.118129
Bad Debt Rate	−.022	1.752198
Long-Term Debt/ Total Assets	5.98	1.456469
Debt Service Coverage	−1.04	2656.429
Fixed Asset Growth	−1.60	5.50693
Return on Assets	1.45	1.449805
Operating Margin	1.56	1.555386
Asset Turnover	1.90	2.501046
Property Plant & Equipment/Beds	−0.64	1.343229
Natural log of Sales	−0.89	1.071831
Net Income/Equity	1.52	4.327021
Net Sales/Total Assets	1.57	4.129053
Long-Term Debt/Equity	−0.95	8.605796
Short-Term Debt/ Total Assets	−8.19	1.352943
Net Working Capital/ Total Assets	0.25	1.187235
Length of Average Patient Stay	−1.34	1.130008
Occupancy Rate	−0.18	1.486862

These changes seem to reflect that the buyer's liquidity ratios would suffer by buying a firm with a weak liquidity position and that debt ratios would increase from borrowing to finance a purchase and by taking over hospitals that had high debt ratios themselves. Also, net income of the parent suffers after the merger largely because of the negative impact of the subsidiary hospital. A summary of the changes in the averages of the ratios one year before merger and one year after merger appears in Table 4.14.

The same t-tests were performed on these variables two years after merger and three years after merger. Again, the values for the variables were compared to these values one year prior to the

TABLE 4.14. Changes in Ratio Averages: One Year Before Merger versus One Year After Merger

Variable	Before Merger	After Merger
Current Ratio	3.33	2.61
Acid Test Ratio	1.62	0.90
Days in Accounts Receivable	73.66	81.76
Bad Debt Rate	5.38%	5.59%
Long-Term Debt/ Total Assets	36.80%	36.46%
Debt Service Coverage	9.07	121.01
Fixed Asset Growth	19.03%	32.16%
Return on Assets	12.94%	8.25%
Operating Margin	6.89%	2.90%
Asset Turnover	1.36	1.14
Property Plant and Equipment/Beds	$116,601	$126,420
Natural log of Sales	17.98	18.20
Net Income/Equity	13.51%	−0.70%
Net Sales/Total Assets	$170.74	$135.23
Long-Term Debt/Equity	107.89%	168.83%
Short-Term Debt/ Total Assets	18.13%	18.31%
Net Working Capital/ Total Assets	22.66%	21.49%
Length of Average Patient Stay	5.51 days	5.92 days
Occupancy Rate	62%	62.82%

merger. Results of the tests comparing the ratios before merger and two years after the merger gave the results shown in Table 4.15.

INTERPRETATION OF THE DATA

1. The merger had a negative impact upon *debt and liquidity ratios*. The long-term debt/equity ratio was severely impacted, which may arise because of the financing of the merger or the taking on of the debt of the subsidiary by the parent causing the combined statements to show very poor debt/equity positions.

2. *Return on equity* (net income/equity) ratio was negatively impacted. Both of these ratios were shown to be the most significant according to their F-values (143 and 124, respectively).

3. *Liquidity ratios*. Current ratio (from an average of 3.33 to an average of 2.49) and acid test ratio (from an average of 1.62 to an average of 0.85) were significant. Thus, comparing the results of the tests on the average of these 19 ratios taken the year before merger and comparing them to averages one and two years after merger gives some predictable results and some consistent results. In both cases, the current ratio and acid test ratio were significantly impacted, with both being lower than their premerger averages.

4. *Leverage ratios*. Debt service coverage was more significantly impacted one year after merger than two years after merger.

5. *Return on equity and debt to equity*. Net income/equity and long-term debt/equity both became more severely affected two years after merger rather than one year after merger. Most other factors were not significantly affected either one year or two years after merger.

As a final analysis, the same tests were performed using data on the same hospitals three years after the merger. Table 4.16 summarizes the findings obtained.

As shown in Table 4.16, effects on values of certain ratios have been consistent and lasting over the three-year period after merger. Once again, the ratios that have shown significant difference three

TABLE 4.15. Changes in Ratio Averages: One Year Before Merger versus Two Years After Merger

Factor	VALUES		F-value	T-value
	Before Merger	2 Years After Merger		
Current Ratio	3.33	2.49	7.937503	0.93
Acid Test Ratio	1.62	0.85	8.841789	0.93
Days in Accounts Receivable	73.66	79.09	1.063315	−0.72
Bad Debt Rate	5.38%	4.62%	2.307851	0.70
Long-Term Debt/ Total Assets	36.80%	37.71%	1.860795	−0.13
Debt Service Coverage	9.07	9.51	5.524778	−0.08
Fixed Asset Growth	19.03%	18.49%	1.58115	0.11
Return on Assets	12.94%	8.74%	1.100351	1.11
Operating Margin	6.89%	3.28%	1.420322	1.23
Asset Turnover	1.36	1.20	2.800015	1.21
Property Plant and Equipment/Beds	111,601	126,184	2.41046	−0.60
Natural log of Sales	17.98	18.11	1.07154	−0.48
Net Income/Equity	13.51%	−61.19%	124.4677	1.69
Net Sales/Total Assets	170.74%	148.92%	2.741155	0.81
Long-Term Debt/Equity	107.89%	476.45%	143.5291	−1.51
Short-Term Debt/ Total Assets	18.13%	19.81%	1.664268	−0.61
Net Working Capital/ Total Assets	22.66%	18.78%	1.105277	0.70
Length of Average Patient Stay	5.51 days	5.83 days	1.211287	−1.02
Occupancy Rate	62.0%	63.1%	2.838004	−0.23

TABLE 4.16. Changes in Ratio Averages: One Year Before Merger versus Three Years After Merger

Factor	VALUES		F-value	T-value
	Before Merger	3 Years After Merger		
Current Ratio	3.33	2.48	7.920402	0.97
Acid Test Ratio	1.62	1.00	7.787471	0.74
Days in Accounts Receivable	73.66 days	76.2 days	1.292123	−0.36
Bad Debt Rate	5.38%	5.65%	1.980771	−0.25
Long-Term Debt/ Total Assets	36.80%	37.45%	1.175488	−0.11
Debt Service Coverage	9.07	3.65	16.98911	2.03
Fixed Asset Growth	19.03	23.69	1.990617	−0.78
Return on Assets	12.94%	8.88%	1.380732	1.14
Operating Margin	6.89%	2.92%	1.170027	1.52
Asset Turnover	1.36	1.14	2.55743	1.71
Property Plant and Equipment/Beds	116,601	138,855	1.652417	−1.37
Natural log of Sales	17.98	18.25	1.141136	−1.04
Net Income/Equity	13.51%	10.91%	2.28513	0.45
Net Sales/Total Assets	170.74%	144.91%	2.225339	0.97
Long-Term Debt/Equity	107.89%	213.44%	24.10301	−1.02
Short-Term Debt/ Total Assets	18.13%	18.11%	1.227465	1.02
Net Working Capital/ Total Assets	22.66%	18.15%	1.153684	0.87
Length of Average Patient Stay	5.51 days	5.81 days	1.170331	−0.97
Occupancy Rate	62.0%	62.93%	1.204757	−0.18

years after merger include the debt and liquidity ratios. The long-term debt/equity ratio has increased by a factor of almost two and is shown to be the most significant change over the period (F-value of 24).

The factor with the second highest F-value is the debt service coverage ratio (reducing from 9.07 premerger to an average of 3.65 three years after merger). Again, this result may be from the acquiring hospital taking on more debt to finance the purchase and/or the acquiring firm assuming much of the debt of their subsidiary. As in the other two years after merger, the liquidity ratios of current ratio and acid test ratio are significantly below those of the premerger amounts or values. It is interesting to note that the profitability ratios (most noteworthy, the net income/equity ratio) have stabilized three years after merger and their differences with the premerger values are no longer considered significant. The remaining ratios show no significant variations.

SUMMARY OF VARIABLES BY SOURCE

The results of this study offer some insight into the effects of hospital mergers and the characteristics of hospitals sought for merger during the 1980s in California. An interesting comparison of the results given above with the results of previous studies (Simkowitz and Monroe, 1971; Singh, 1971; Stevens, 1973; Wansley and Lane, 1984; Wansley, 1984) shows differences and similarities. These studies had been performed most often on Fortune 500 firms in specific industries, but none were done on the hospital industry. Many of these studies and their results were presented in the literature review in Chapter 2.

The results of these studies was compared with the findings of this study. Studies done in the period 1969 to the mid-1980s concentrated on the isolation of those variables that separated target firms versus nontarget firms. Later studies (Omurtak, 1986; Mullner and Anderson, 1987; McCue, McCue, and Wheeler, 1988) extended this early work to include the accuracy of models to predict takeover targets based on financial and accounting data. Thus, earlier studies offered the factors that were considered significant in takeovers with no predictive analysis. The following summary will attempt to compare the results of early and more recent works with the results found in this work. Again, what separates this work from others is the inclusion of classifications of merged and nonmerged firms and the industry-specific analysis, which was not performed until recently.

REFERENCE NOTES

1. *Individual Hospital Financial Data for California June 30, 1989-June 29, 1990*, Office of Statewide Health Planning and Development, Sacramento CA. June 1991, vi.

2. Michael Simkowitz and Robert J. Monroe, "A Discriminant Analysis Function for Conglomerate Targets," *The Southern Journal of Business*, November 1971, 1-16.

3. Donald L. Stevens, "Financial Characteristics of Merged Firms: A Multivariate Analysis," *Journal of Financial and Quantitative Analysis*, March 1973, 149-158.

4. James W. Wansley and William R. Lane, "A Financial Profile of Merged Firms," *Review of Business & Economic Research*, Fall 1984, 87-98.

5. Number Crunching Statistical System Version 5.01.

6. Number Crunching Statistical System version 5.01 *Reference Manual*, 1989, 133.

7. Variable fixed asset growth was not considered significant in the model one year prior to merger. Thus, it was not included in further analyses.

Chapter 5

Marketing and Operational Factors That Affect the Success of Mergers and Acquisitions

MARKET SHARE

Most hospital mergers are contemplated in order to increase a competitive advantage. Managers hope that market share will increase for the new organization in comparison to the shares previously held. Because increases in market share improve an organization's competitive position, a snowball effect can occur. However, market share alone does not mandate success. Without sound management, a merger has a high probability of failure.

COMPATIBILITY AND CONFLICT OF SERVICES

It is rare for two organizations not to have overlapping services or markets. The usual strategy is to eliminate the least efficient and consolidate services geographically. Often the weaker unit will leave the acute care field in favor of long-term care or outpatient services. In developing a market analysis of the prospective merger candidates, this factor is usually considered a positive point. Of course, caution is necessary: two units with similar services may be in direct conflict when management styles, labor relations, and physician loyalty is analyzed.

THE CHANGING ROLE
OF CENTERS OF EXCELLENCE

A few years ago, a hospital was known by its centers of excellence, and there still are a few that stake their reputation on this strategy. Such centers are not what they once were. A brief history is needed to bring us up to date. Here are a few citations that tell the story.

An article in *Hospitals*[1] discusses how the concept is successfully applied in hospitals around the country. In one study, ". . . 57 percent of hospital CEOs reported that they had designated one or more services as a priority program. Approximately 44 percent reported that they had selected three or more programs for development."[2]

Magnet Hospitals Were Predecessors to Rational Centers

A two-part article in *JONA* discusses the concept of the Magnet Hospital. While the emphasis of the article is on nursing, the authors make the point that such hospitals maintain staffing levels even during shortages.[3]

A Center May Have a Better Reputation
Than Its Parent Hospital

An article in the *Journal of Health Care Marketing*[4] offers a methodology to increase hospital revenue through the use of such centers with a direct approach to potential patients. The article cites various studies that review hospital selection for different services, and the highest patient selection rates were in women's services.[5]

The article noted that centers of excellence and the hospitals that sponsor them may have greater approval ratings in the eyes of the public.[6]

Barich and Kotler[7] encourage organizations to track their images and take steps to achieve or maintain a positive image. They state that each image factor is made up of a number of attributes among which are products (or services) offered.

Such characteristics as the quality and reliability of a service are cited as directly affecting this image. It is obvious that well-respected centers of excellence positively affect image and therefore revenues.

Centers Will Help Hospitals to Continue to Prosper

This point of view—that centers of excellence are needed for hospitals to continue to prosper—is discussed by Jeff Goldsmith.[8] Goldsmith makes three points:

1. Hospitals are more than merely businesses.[9] In effect, he supports the inclusion of Core Values in the mission statement.
2. He states that hospitals should have a new mission to treat those with chronic problems.
3. Another point that Goldsmith makes is that doctors remain at the center of health care delivery and that hospitals will continue to find it essential to collaborate with doctors in providing care for the community.[10]

Forming a Joint Center

Sheldon S. King of Cedars-Sinai Medical Center of Los Angeles[11] found it beneficial to cooperate with UCLA Medical Center to avoid unnecessary competition and thereby serve the region more appropriately by focusing on services each center is best at providing. King also stated that hospitals should provide community services such as access to proper housing, adequate nutrition, and psychological counseling after discharge from the hospital.

Forming a Rural Network to Create Excellence

John D. Hicks, CEO of North Mississippi Medical Center[12] restructured his hospital by developing a network of seven rural hospitals. Previous to this effort he had merged two hospital-based ambulance services together in order to provide better service. In this situation, Hicks converted county owned hospitals into a private, not-for-profit healthcare network. In Lee county, hospital managers wanted the hospital to grow while the county officials were not interested in expansion. He bought the hospital's assets from the county for $25 million and restructured obsolete hospitals into a network that meets the needs of today's rural Mississippi residents.

Humana Uses the Centers of Excellence Concept as a Corporate Strategy

Humana Corporation[13] began developing its Centers for Excellence program in 1982. As of 1988, 17 of Humana's 25 hospitals had such centers. The centers are designed to increase admissions and prestige. Since a large patient base is required for a center, they are limited to large, metropolitan facilities. The centers also help enhance physicians' practices.

Joint Ventures Strengthen Ties to Docs

Torrence (California) Memorial Medical Center divested itself of four of its major outpatient services to a for-profit joint venture with its medical staff. The new entity, Health Access Systems, averted competition from members of the medical staff, expanded market share, increased revenue, and built a well-capitalized base for further ventures. By providing more than one service, the new corporation had a major competitive advantage.[14]

New forms of competition have forced changes in the concept. Excellence is being defined as regional quality. A center of excellence needs to have a regional market or an even larger market. Within that expanded market, the center must be know for its exceptional quality.

Unfortunately, quality is a difficult concept to define. The quantitative form of quality has adherents who have developed awards for excellence in various fields, e.g., risk management.[15] The leading example is Daniel Freeman Hospitals in Inglewood and Marina Del Rey, California. By bringing their program in-house, they reduced litigation and cut costs. Other examples cited involved a surgi-center, and an out-patient clinic. One result was better communications between HMO managers and their customers.

Internal definitions of quality often are hollow marketing ploys. Multiplying awards for quality offers even marginal providers the certainty of winning awards in both operations and marketing.[16]

Quality is more than good numbers. It must include a patient satisfaction program that goes below surface features and provides true excellence in care. Warm food and a short response time to a call button may be far more valuable than any award.

With downsizing and reframing required because of reduced reimbursement, ensuring quality is ever more important and also more difficult. We must learn to trim without decreasing the quality of patient care and negatively influencing customer satisfaction. We acknowledge that this is much easier to say than to do.

Creativity and inclusiveness are the keys to quality improvement. At a recent seminar that Dr. Goldman conducted, one of the participants asked if employees with menial jobs should be included in the planning process. The group's response was that they also see what customers need and want and can make excellent contributions in both customer satisfaction and increased efficiency.

Customer empowerment is also a tool to better quality. Some acute care patients are healthier than others. By authorizing customers to get their own extra towels or authorized snacks, nursing time can be used more efficiently and the patients will feel more self-sufficient.

We say that centers of excellence must be excellent. They must fit into your strategic plan and be more than a promotional tool. With the current era of ever-increasing competition, nothing less will do.

MANAGED CARE

Managed care will not disappear. Instead, it will change the map of health care. Where once poorly performing hospitals closed, the need to capture market share, expand into new markets, and become more efficient in order to obtain contracts will force mergers and acquisitions.

Several surveys conducted a few years ago predicted high levels of closures. Yet follow-up research showed that about half, or even less, of the hospitals predicted to close were forced to do so.[17]

Hospitals are merging rather than closing[18] and part of the reason is that managed care organizations want to contract with networks that offer good geographical coverage. Some experts question the value of such mergers by raising the issues of who will benefit from them. Will these new, stronger organizations use their increased market power to support their charitable and educational missions or will they raise prices?[19]

A related question is how well the newer organizations can bargain with their managed care foes. They may gain regional coverage by acquiring marginal hospitals. Yet, these hospitals may reduce efficiency and cause operational problems. It may be a better strategy to affiliate with these hospitals rather than absorbing them.

Managed care will also modify how and where services are offered. If, for example, a center of excellence attracts patients exclusively from the hospital's primary service area, there is little prospect for additional reimbursement as a "Carve-Out" under a full risk contract. Instead of bringing new revenue from new patients, a weak center that is not accepted for regional use will add costs.

Under full-risk contracts, hospitals and physicians are required to provide a set of services. But, they have the option of providing them in their own way. If a center encourages people to increase their use of the service the center offers, costs go up while revenue remains the same.

Carve-Outs are the answer. True centers of excellence may be part of an organization's merger and acquisition strategy. Increased patient use will increase the quality of care and enable the network to obtain service-based contracts. A regional cardiac surgery program benefits because a separate contract offers additional reimbursement.

RESTRUCTURING SERVICES TO FIT THE NEW ORGANIZATION

Mergers and acquisitions force the restructuring of services in the name of increased efficiency and better customer service. Services are introduced, modified, or eliminated to meet the needs of the new organization and the markets it is trying to capture.

However, decisions are sometimes based on inadequate or faulty analytical techniques and erroneous assumptions. We know that since the advent of the Prospective Payment Reimbursement approach, hospitals have been forced to cut unprofitable services. Even when such a strategy is in conflict with the hospital's mission statement, service elimination often proceeds with the justification that the hospital must survive.

Although the pressure on health service institutions to cut costs, either by eliminating services or downsizing operations, is today's reality, some administrators are inherently inclined toward eliminating services and scaling down operations based on their belief that profitability is the sole objective. In opposition to this contention, many health service professionals believe that services should be continued even if unprofitable, as long as the institution can support it from Cash Cows. They argue that service to the community should take precedence over profits. However, with managed care contributing an increasing percentage of business, retaining a marginal service may increase costs with little or no effect on revenues.

If a service must be eliminated, Managed Service Restructuring (MSR) provides the procedures to avoid unwarranted reduction or alteration, and are the least damaging to the institution and to the public. Such an analysis can be the basis of a realignment plan that can satisfy all parties–the community, the medical staff, the organization's employees and its administrators–and must be included in all analyses of potential mergers or acquisitions.

The worst time to make a restructuring decision is when a crisis arises. Early detection of problems is critical. The symptoms that indicate an impending crisis include the following situations:

- the demand for the service is declining at an increasing rate
- maintaining the current level of revenue requires an increase in promotional activities
- the number of employees per unit of service is rising
- related services are also experiencing one or more of the above symptoms
- demographic or competitive changes are resulting in these symptoms

In other words, the service appears to have become a "Dog." However, an analysis using the MSR format determines the actual situation and leads to a positive solution.

Applying MSR

Managed Service Restructuring is a conscious management effort to retain a seemingly unprofitable existing service. The service may appear to be unprofitable for either the short- or long-run. The service may be altered or moved to another institution. The need for MSR may arise either due to changes in demand, inadequate management, or the structure of the new organization.

The MSR technique is most profitably used when management is unable to identify the stages of a service's life cycle, or to recognize the service's place in the new organization's portfolio. However, our contention is that MSR be considered in all situations involving the possibility of any health service elimination.

The basis for this contention is that:

1. Health service involves public service; it concerns the health and welfare of human beings.
2. Restructuring involves analysis to determine whether a profitable means of salvaging the service exists and allows the institution to re-evaluate its financial and marketing strategies.
3. Restructuring avoids elimination based on erroneous assumptions and theoretical bias.

Downsizing May Increase the Decline

Postmerger downsizing may, in fact, damage the organization. Many managers now equate service elimination with failure caused by poor planning, poor implementation, or poor management. Often the elimination occurs because of analytical faults or what many call "analysis paralysis." Rather than using downsizing as a strategy, one can apply the MSR technique. One important principle is to *not make enemies by accident.* That is, the course of action to be taken should acknowledge and address the needs and sensibilities of the hospital's publics–patients, medical staff, families, employees, governments, and community.

MSR Techniques

First, carry out an analysis of the financial and market factors and establish whether the service is in fact a Dog. If analyzing a product or service suggests it is a Dog or in the decline stage, the service may have to be eliminated. However, managers should also consider harvesting (selling off a service to another organization) or modifying the way the service is offered. This is particularly valid after a merger or acquisition.

Finally, if it is determined that the service must be eliminated, the community can be brought into the decision-making process so that they accept the course of action. They will not be happy about the loss of a valued service, but they will have little or no animosity toward the institution or the decision makers. When a large network acquires a small, community hospital, the need is especially great to gain the confidence of the new community.

The development of a community advisory board and the holding of community meetings to explain the problem and listen to alternatives can build goodwill. Of course, an open mind is essential. Ground rules can be stated. The community members will accept the concept that change must occur in order to maintain the overall health of the institution.

If the service is slated to be transferred or sold off to a competitor, a complete analysis may find that the service in question is declining because a competitor is increasing market share. A competitor may be willing and capable of ensuring the continuity of the service.

The service may also be restructured or rebuilt within the organization. It may be moved from an inpatient to an outpatient setting or from one facility to another. The number of employees may be reduced. Promotion can be increased, reorganized, or reduced. Pricing may also be realigned. The objective, under this option, is to increase usage or users.

As a broad and general guideline, MSR may be applied as follows:

Options	Conditions
1. Selling off	All other options considered inappropriate.
2. Selling off to a competitor	Dwindling demand is the result of the rising market share of the competition and the organization is unable to regain market share.
3. Product life cycle and status	Rebuild within the organization of the service identified, restructuring found feasible after marketing and financial analysis.
4. Joint Venture	This provides a source of financing and expertise for reorganization.

A "Dog" could be continued as long as it shows some profit. However, the MSR strategy suggests that a proper analysis of profit or loss of a service requires that expenses and revenues be meticulously isolated. This is essential because a decline in demand of one service may affect the demand of another related service.

The MSR strategy requires an examination of alternate restructuring options including realignment, increased promotion, managed divestiture, and community involvement before service termination. Restructuring can lead to future expansion and profitability. Such actions also improve the public image of the organization. In any situation involving service reconsideration, the MSR strategy is a viable alternative to immediate elimination of the service or product line.

OPERATIONAL FACTORS

Staffing Issues

In addition to compatibility problems between the newly joined medical staffs, there well may be labor issues as involved. Lyncheski and McDermott[20] recommend conducting an audit to avoid problems in the following areas:

- Employee handbooks and policy manuals
- All employee physician and independent service contracts
- Product life cycle and status
- Part-time staffing arrangements
- Fringe benefits for both full-time and part-time employees, particularly those that might "guarantee" lifetime or retirement benefits
- Accrued but unpaid obligations relating to wages, vacation pay, and taxes
- Workers' and unemployment compensation

They recommend developing an element within your merger or acquisition plan that consists of two parts:

1. Integration of the two organizations from the labor and employment perspective
2. Communication to employees, customers, and the community[21]

Physical Plants

The physical plants of the new organization may be incompatible from a marketing perspective and may also cause problems between staffs. Despite the quality of care provided, if a building looks outdated or dilapidated, there will be a perception of low quality.

We have seen medical staffs and employees from the more attractive facility refuse to cooperate with their counterparts at the other one. Two examples should be sufficient: (1) transfers between compatible units in the two hospitals are sabotaged, and (2) physicians from the more attractive hospital have considered the peers at the other hospital to be less competent.

Of course, these considerations must be included in the merger or acquisition plan. Upgrading the less attractive facility as well as coordinating signage, etc., must be included in the merger or acquisition budget.

REFERENCE NOTES

1. Therese Droste, " 'Center of Excellence' Name Tag Carries Clout," *Hospitals*, July 20, 1989, 54.

2. Ibid.

3. Marlene Kramer and Claudia Schmalenberg, "Magnet Hospitals, Parts I and II, Institutions of Excellence," *JONA*, Vol. 18, No. 1. Jan. 1988, 13 ff. and Vol. 18, No. 2, 11 ff.

4. Scot M. Smith and Marta Clark, "Hospital Image and the Positioning of Service Centers: An Application in Market Analysis and Strategy Development," *Journal of Health Care Marketing*, Vol. 10, No. 3, September 1990, 12-22.

5. Op. Cit., 13.

6. Ibid.

7. Howard Barich and Philip Kotler, "A Framework for Marketing Image Management," *Sloan Management Review*, Vol. 32, No. 2, Winter, 1991, p. 94 ff.

8. Jeff Goldsmith, "A Radical Prescription for Hospitals," *Harvard Business Review*, May-June 1989, 104-111.

9. Op. Cit., 105.

10. Op. Cit., 107-108.

11. Steve Taravelia, "Defining the Hospital's Role: New CEO Expands Mission Beyond Healthcare," *Modern Healthcare*, December 8, 1989, 54.

12. Sandy Lutz, "Planting the Seeds of Growth: He Turned One Hospital into a Rural Network," *Modern Healthcare*, May 12, 1989, 48.

13. Cynthia Wallace, "Centers for Excellence: Humana Hopes to Gain Prestige as Well as More Hospital Inpatients from Its Medical Specialty Centers," *Modern Healthcare*, May 20, 1988, 30.

14. Sally Berger, "Hospital Strengthens Ties to Doctors with Joint Venture," *Modern Healthcare*, January 29, 1988, 39.

15. "Looking Beyond Acute Care," *Modern Healthcare*, October 24, 1994, 56 ff.

16. "Everyone's a Winner," *Modern Healthcare*, August 22, 1994, 26 ff.

17. "As Closure Forecasters, Administrators Rate Poor," *Modern Healthcare*, July 6, 1992, 20.

18. "Hospitals Now Merge Rather Than Close," *Modern Healthcare*, July 6, 1992, 30 ff.

19. "Panel Asks Who Gains in Hospital Mergers," *Modern Healthcare*, November 28, 1994, 10.

20. John E. Lyncheski and Joseph M. McDermott, "Labor Issues Can Hinder Hospital Mergers," *HR Magazine*, September 1993, 70.

21. Ibid., 71.

Chapter 6

Postmerger Analysis

In an attempt to determine the success of the hospital mergers in this study, analysis was performed on the merged hospitals three years after the mergers. This allows sufficient time for the merged entity to show improved or lower ratios. To perform this comparative analysis, the mergers were divided into successful and unsuccessful categories depending on the changes in the significant variables from the year of merger to three years after merger.

The significant ratios chosen were:

- current ratio
- acid test ratio
- debt service coverage ratio
- fixed asset growth
- net income/equity
- net sales/total assets
- long-term debt/equity

These were the variables that significantly changed for the parent company one year before merger compared to one year after merger. They are discussed and illustrated in Chapter 4. The significant ratios that divide targeted hospitals from nontargeted hospitals one year prior to merger were current ratio, bad debt ratio, long-term debt/total assets, return on assets, operating margin, net income/equity, and short-term debt/total assets. These were also discussed in Chapter 4.

To separate successful and unsuccessful mergers three years after the merger, liquidity (measured by current and acid test ratios), profitability (measured by net income/equity and net income/total assets), and debt ratios (measured by long-term debt/equity) were calculated. Tables 6.1 and 6.2 list the successful and unsuccessful mergers by name.

Table 6.3 illustrates the changes in values of the ratios of the parent hospital one year before to three years after the merger.

It can be seen from the numbers that liquidity has been adversely affected. The current ratio and acid test ratio on the average declined by 1.77 and 1.14, respectively. Also, profitability has decreased from 10.34 percent to 2.24 percent, a measure by net income divided by equity. Finally, the debt portion of the merged firms has greatly increased. As measured by long-term debt divided by equity, the change has been from 118 percent to 278 percent. Table 6.4 illustrates the changes in the same ratios for successful mergers.

In these situations, the liquidity ratios of the merged hospitals have increased and the profitable ratio, net income/ equity, has increased by more than five times. But, even though these show improved

TABLE 6.1. Successful Mergers

Purchased Hospital	Parent
Santa Rosa General Hospital	Santa Rosa Memorial Hospital
Doctor's Hospital of Lakewood Clark Avenue	Doctor's Hospital of Lakewood South Street
Memorial Hospital, Ceres	Memorial Hospital, Modesto
Modesto City Hospital	Doctor's Medical Center
Marshall Hale Hospital	Children's Hospital of San Francisco
Hollywood Presbyterian Hospital	Queen of Angels Medical Center
Dominican Community Hospital of Santa Cruz	Dominican Santa Cruz Hospital
Ontario Community Hospital	Doctor's Hospital of Montclair
Doctor's Hospital of Santa Ana	Santa Ana Hospital
Alvarado Parkway Hospital	Alvarado Community Hospital

Note: Postmerger names are used throughout because that is how the hospitals are registered with the OSHPD.

TABLE 6.2. Unsuccessful Mergers

Purchased Hospital	Parent
Sierra Care Hospital	Sonora Community Hospital
Beverly Glen Hospital	Beverly Hills Medical Center
The Garden Campus	California Pacific Medical Center
O'Connor Hospital of Campbell	O'Connor Hospital
Pinecrest Hospital	Santa Barbara Cottage Hospital
Riverside Community Hospital Knollwood Center	Riverside Community Hospital
Community Hospital Recovery Center	Community Hospital of the Monterey Peninsula
Simi Valley Community Hospital	Simi Valley Adventist Hospital
Ukiah General Hospital	Ukiah Adventist Hospital
Peralta Hospital	Samuel Merritt Hospital
Herrick Hospital Health Center	Alta Bates Hospital
Mission Oakes Hospital	Good Samaritan of Santa Clara
Lodi Memorial Hospital-West	Lodi Memorial Hospital
Mission Hospital	Community Hospital, Huntington Park
Van Nuys Community Hospital	Hollywood Community Hospital
Providence Hospital	Merritt Hospital

Note: Postmerger names are used throughout because that is how the hospitals are registered with the OSHPD.

positions, the long-term debt/equity has increased substantially, but most of that is due to a single merge. Thus, even for mergers that can be classified as successful, the debt position of the merged hospitals is still very adversely affected three years after the merger.

In an attempt to see if successful and unsuccessful mergers can be predicted or identified before the merger takes place, information was gathered concerning the hospitals that were targeted in these mergers. That data was presented in an earlier chapter in an attempt to predict takeover targets. At this time, that information regarding the targeted hospitals can be separated into two categories. The first category consists of targeted hospitals that resulted in unsuccessful

TABLE 6.3. Changes in Values of the Ratios of Parent Hospitals

Factor	Before Merger	After Merger	Difference
Current Ratio	3.82	2.05	(1.77)
Acid Test Ratio	1.68	0.54	(1.14)
Debt Service Coverage	6.59	3.41	(3.18)
Fixed Asset Growth	19.49	13.67	(5.82)
Net Income/Equity	10.34%	2.24%	(8.10%)
Net Sales/Total Assets	153.55%	162.22%	+8.67%
Long-Term Debt/Equity	117.53%	278.17%	+160.64%

TABLE 6.4. Changes in Same Ratios for Successful Mergers

Factor	Before Merger	After Merger	Difference
Current Ratio	2.55	3.03	+0.48
Acid Test Ratio	0.51	0.83	+0.32
Debt Service Coverage	12.31	352.75	+340.44
Fixed Asset Growth	18.31	17.32	(0.99)
Net Income/Equity	18.56%	101.97%	+83.41%
Net Sales/Total Assets	198.27%	218.11%	+19.84%
Long-Term Debt/Equity	92.51%	1,018.54%	+926.03%

Note: The long-term debt/equity change was drastically affected by one outlier. If that outlier had not been included, the ratio would be 44.40.

mergers. The second group consists of targeted hospitals that resulted in successful mergers. The same seven variables that were found to be significant in differentiating targeted and nontargeted hospitals are used here. The ratios used:

- current ratio
- bad debt ratio

- long term debt/total assets
- return on assets
- operating margin
- net income/equity
- short-term debt/total assets

These were found to be significant in predicting takeover targets with similar rates of approximately 90 percent for one year before merger (see Chapter 4).

The averages of the ratios for targeted firms that resulted in unsuccessful mergers versus the ratios for those targets that resulted in successful mergers are given in Table 6.5.

From the absolute numbers, some large differences can be seen. In general, it appears that the target hospitals that resulted in a successful merger had a better liquid position (measured by higher current ratios), were more profitable (measured by higher return on assets, operating margins, and net income/equity percentages), had less long-term debt (measured by long-term debt/total asset percentages), and a bit more relative short-term debt. These would seem to be reasonable expectations for an entity looking to buy another.

In order to test whether these differences in the target hospitals were significant, a discriminant analysis was performed in the ratios of these two groups. The results of that analysis are shown in Table 6.6.

TABLE 6.5

Factor	Unsuccessful	Successful	Differences
Current Ratio	1.81	2.31	+0.50
Bad Debt Ratio	7.13%	8.20%	+1.07%
Long-Term Debt/ Total Assets	42.40%	32.91%	(9.29%)
Return on Assets	(6.49%)	(3.41%)	+3.08%
Operating Margin	(14.28%)	(6.22%)	+8.06%
Net Income/Equity	(85.81%)	(21.33%)	+64.48%
Short-Term Debt/ Total Assets	42.35%	45.27%	+2.92%

According to Table 6.6, none of the variables is significant in differentiating or predicting successful and unsuccessful mergers. These were the same variables that were significant in predicting takeover targets. The overall Wilk's lambda for this function was 0.8286. It appears that the same variables that the model found to be significant for parents targeting firms for takeover are no longer significant in determining the success of the merger three years later. This could mean that the wrong variables are being considered when trying to find proper targeted hospitals. Also, the success rate of properly classifying firms as leading to success or not was not significant. Table 6.7 summarizes the success rate of proper classification. The success ratios are approximately 50 percent—no better than flipping a coin.

TABLE 6.6. Weight and Significance of Variables of Targeted Hospitals

Factor	Unsuccessful	Successful	Differences
Current Ratio	2.562318	2.505186	0.0
Bad Debt Ratio	(0.005429)	(0.006561)	0.0
Long-Term Debt/ Total Assets	0.088076	0.088980	1.4
Return on Assets	0.3020253	0.2016979	0.0
Operating Margin	(0.528420)	(0.405287)	0.011
Net Income/Equity	0.013302	0.014355	0.047
Short-Term Debt/ Total Assets	0.1014237	0.1029097	0.001

TABLE 6.7. Predictive Success Rate Three Years After Merger

Factor	Successful Merger	Unsuccessful Merger
Predicted to be successful	6	8
Predicted to be unsuccessful	4	8
Total	10	16
Success rate	60%	50%

To summarize, there are significant differences between hospitals that were targeted as acquisitions and those not targeted. Those differences dealt with relative liquidity, profitability, and debt positions. When analyzing the results of the merger three years later, it is found that those same significant variables that separated targeted and nontargeted hospitals do not offer any significant predictive information regarding the success of the parent organization. Further work needs to be done in this area both by hospital administrators and researchers to attempt to identify the characteristics of targeted firms that lead to success years later.

Chapter 7

Recommendations and Conclusions

We performed a final analysis to determine whether there were any differences in the targeted financial firms' positions prior to takeover that lead to successful or unsuccessful mergers. We employed all 19 ratios that were previously employed in our study to discriminate between targeted and nontargeted organizations one last time.

Previous results found that seven ratios were able to significantly separate the two groups. They were:

- current ratio
- bad debt rate
- long-term debt/total assets
- return on assets
- operating margin
- net income/equity
- short-term debt/total assets

After this final analysis, using all 19 ratios, we found *only one* variable that was statistically significant when predicting successful and unsuccessful mergers or acquisitions. As you will see in Table 7.1, it was more useful as a warning tool than a predictor of success.

This predictor is *net sales/total assets*. Fortunately, this is a logical variable and the logical conclusion is that hospitals that are efficiently and aggressively using their assets to increase sales, will probably succeed after the merger.

The F-value associated with this ratio was 6.3. No other variable has an F-value of more than one. The overall Wilk's Lambda was 0.7863. The absolute values for this ratio averaged 203.11 percent for targeted firms leading to successful mergers and 127.20 percent for those leading to unsuccessful takeovers. Liquidity, profitability, and debt position were found to have no significant difference between the two groups.

By employing only one ratio—one that is easy to rapidly calculate from published data—the predictive ability of the model is useful as shown in Table 7.1.

By using this ratio, managers can be warned of potentially unsuccessful situations and delve further into marketing and operational factors to improve the total analysis.

It seems, therefore, that in a practical model for managing the merger/acquisition process, we must also rely on nonfinancial factors to obtain success in these situations. That is, the marketing mix between the two entities must make sense or the new venture will—at the minimum—be in serious trouble. The new organization may be so financially burdened that it will be crippled for many years.

Successful organizations must make human resource and operational sense. They must increase the organization's capacity to compete in its current markets, permit it to enter new markets, help it develop new products, or allow it to diversify into other fields.

In conclusion, the competitive forces of *the current* health care marketplace dictate that every management tool must be applied to the merger or acquisition situation. Successful firms will not stop at just a financial analysis or merely a marketing analysis. Instead, they will take operational, human resource, financial, and marketing factors into consideration. Most important, they will view the coupling in light of community needs.

TABLE 7.1. Prediction Success Rate Three Years After Merger

Factor	Successful Merger	Unsuccessful Merger
Predicted to be successful	5	4
Predicted to be unsuccessful	5	12
Total	10	16
Success rate	50%	75%

Appendix A

Variable Names

	Merged Firms	Nonmerged Firms
Current Ratio	C1	C21
Acid Test Ratio	C2	C22
Days in Accounts Receivable	C3	C23
Bad Debt Rate	C4	C24
Long-Term Debt/Total Assets	C5	C25
Debt Service Coverage	C6	C26
Fixed Asset Growth	C7	C27
Return on Assets	C8	C28
Operating Margin	C9	C29
Asset Turnover	C10	C30
Property Plant and Equipment/Beds	C11	C31
Natural Log of Total Revenue	C12	C32
Net Income/Equity	C13	C33
Total Revenue/Total Assets	C14	C34
Long-Term Debt/Equity	C15	C35
Short-Term Debt/Total Assets	C16	C36
Net Working Capital/Total Assets	C17	C37
Length of Patient Stay	C18	C38
Occupancy Rate	C19	C39
Dummy Variable	C20	

Appendix B

Discriminant Analysis of Nineteen Variables One Year, Two Years, Three Years, Four Years, and Five Years Before Merger

Group Counts Report

Group	Count
All	28
1	7
2	21

Variable Selection Report

Classification Variable: C20

In	Variable	R2-Ad	F-Val	F-Prob	R2-Xs	In	Variable	R2-Ad	F-Val	F-Prob	R2-Xs
Yes	C1	0.331	09.9	0.0051	0.6433	Yes	C4	0.245	06.5	0.0192	0.1568
Yes	C5	0.387	12.6	0.0020	0.8880	Yes	C8	0.655	38.0	0.0000	0.9736
Yes	C9	0.601	30.1	0.0000	0.9492	Yes	C13	0.595	29.4	0.0000	0.6167
Yes	C16	0.546	24.0	0.0001	0.7058	No	C2	0.001	0.0	0.9011	0.8733
No	C3	0.034	0.7	0.4249	0.2331	No	C6	0.073	1.5	0.2349	0.7610
No	C7	0.114	2.4	0.1343	0.3630	No	C10	0.073	1.5	0.2363	0.4345
No	C11	0.004	0.1	0.7914	0.5804	No	C12	0.022	0.4	0.5212	0.4912
No	C14	0.003	0.1	0.8215	0.6095	No	C15	0.000	0.0	0.9400	0.5166
No	C17	0.038	0.8	0.3949	0.7443	No	C18	0.061	1.2	0.2820	0.5608
No	C19	0.022	0.4	0.5240	0.6088						

Overall Wilk's Lambda 0.1338

Classification Matrix

Classification Variable: C20
Independent Variables C1 C4 C5 C8 C9 C13 C16
Group Counts Table

	P(All)	P(1)	P(2)
A(All)	47	18	29
A(1)	18	16	2
A(2)	29	2	27

Percent reduction in classification error due to X's 83.0

Linear Discriminant Functions

Classification Variable: C20

Group	1	2
CONSTANT	−97.59063	−44.97266
C1	30.39508	21.58451
C4	−1.020957	−0.3263474
C5	0.4631253	0.2996372
C8	3.872039	2.408948
C9	−5.49326	−3.415032
C13	−0.6900123	−0.3567182
C16	1.910542	1.264753

Misclassified Rows

Row	Act	Pred	P(1)	P(2)
1	1	2	0.000	1.000
22	1	2	0.000	1.000
31	2	1	1.000	0.000
44	2	1	1.000	0.000

Group Counts Report

Group	Count
All	32
1	9
2	23

Variable Selection Report

Classification Variable: C20

In	Variable	R2-Ad	F-Val	F-Prob	R2-Xs	In	Variable	R2-Ad	F-Val	F-Prob	R2-Xs
Yes	C1	0.017	0.4	0.5201	0.3738	Yes	C4	0.067	1.7	0.2030	0.2748
Yes	C5	0.025	0.6	0.4380	0.4240	Yes	C8	0.034	0.9	0.3641	0.9434
Yes	C9	0.030	0.7	0.3967	0.9417	Yes	C13	0.024	0.6	0.4535	0.6276
Yes	C16	0.005	0.1	0.7357	0.7593	No	C2	0.004	0.1	0.7554	0.4985
No	C3	0.005	0.1	0.7282	0.4309	No	C6	0.003	0.1	0.8037	0.5041
No	C7	0.084	2.1	0.1603	0.6031	No	C10	0.128	3.4	0.0785	0.5537
No	C11	0.103	2.6	0.1184	0.1991	No	C12	0.165	4.6	0.0438	0.2397
No	C14	0.055	1.3	0.2597	0.7168	No	C15	0.026	0.6	0.4429	0.7389
No	C17	0.016	0.4	0.5430	0.9698	No	C18	0.000	0.0	0.9284	0.5939
No	C19	0.002	0.0	0.8360	0.4077						

Overall Wilk's Lambda 0.6565

Classification Matrix

Classification Variable: C20
Independent Variables C1 C4 C5 C8 C9 C13 C16
Group Counts Table

	P(All)	P(1)	P(2)
A(All)	48	18	30
A(1)	20	16	4
A(2)	28	2	26

Percent reduction in classification error due to X's 75.0

Linear Discriminant Functions

Classification Variable: C20

Group	1	2
CONSTANT	−6.073441	−6.07499
C1	1.981174	2.364078
C4	0.077044	0.225137
C5	0.045725	0.025464
C8	0.4013201	0.2909721
C9	−0.5346213	−0.3658217
C13	−0.001595	−0.016351
C16	0.077416	0.071684

Misclassified Rows

Row	Act	Pred	P(1)	P(2)
4	1	2	0.398	0.602
5	1	2	0.272	0.728
18	1	2	0.119	0.881
27	1	2	0.352	0.648
41	2	1	0.840	0.160
44	2	1	0.981	0.019

Group Counts Report

Group	Count
All	31
1	10
2	21

Variable Selection Report

Classification Variable: C20

IN	Variable	R2-Ad	F-Val	F-Prob	R2-Xs	IN	Variable	R2-Ad	F-Val	F-Prob	R2-Xs
Yes	C1	0.097	2.5	0.1289	0.4187	Yes	C4	0.104	2.7	0.1156	0.2795
Yes	C5	0.030	0.7	0.4047	0.4717	Yes	C8	0.017	0.4	0.5329	0.9170
Yes	C9	0.002	0.0	0.8448	0.9183	Yes	C13	0.067	1.6	0.2131	0.2683
Yes	C16	0.041	1.0	0.3331	0.4806	No	C2	0.000	0.0	0.9833	0.5059
No	C3	0.101	2.5	0.1304	0.2500	No	C6	0.017	0.4	0.5443	0.7831
No	C7	0.205	5.7	0.0265	0.1771	No	C10	0.043	1.0	0.3301	0.7132
No	C11	0.066	1.6	0.2252	0.3992	No	C12	0.057	1.3	0.2631	0.3673
No	C14	0.000	0.0	0.9577	0.6747	No	C15	0.048	1.1	0.3022	0.9217
No	C17	0.001	0.0	0.8775	0.9482	No	C18	0.009	0.2	0.6666	0.3141
No	C19	0.008	0.2	0.6707	0.3186						

Overall Wilk's Lambda 0.6721

Classification Matrix

Classification Variable: C20
Independent Variables C1 C4 C5 C8 C9 C13 C16
Group Counts Table

	P(All)	P(1)	P(2)
A(All)	45	19	26
A(1)	19	13	6
A(2)	26	6	20

Percent reduction in classification error due to X's 46.7

Linear Discriminant Functions

Classification Variable: C20

Group	1	2
CONSTANT	−6.631062	−8.999908
C1	2.043135	2.676359
C4	0.4745748	0.6894092
C5	0.092672	0.069227
C8	0.2145794	0.2848477
C9	−0.2994441	−0.2649512
C13	−0.000559	−0.007397
C16	0.062560	0.075374

Misclassified Rows

Row	Act	Pred	P(1)	P(2)
1	1	2	0.324	0.676
5	1	2	0.310	0.690
8	1	2	0.498	0.502
13	1	2	0.190	0.810
17	1	2	0.052	0.948
26	1	2	0.447	0.553
30	2	1	1.000	0.000
33	2	1	0.870	0.130
36	2	1	0.905	0.095
40	2	1	0.848	0.152
42	2	1	0.783	0.217
52	2	1	0.659	0.341

Group Counts Report

Group	Count
All	33
1	12
2	21

Variable Selection Report

Classification Variable: C20

IN	Variable	R2-Ad	F-Val	F-Prob	R2-Xs	IN	Variable	R2-Ad	F-Val	F-Prob	R2-Xs
Yes	C1	0.031	0.8	0.3803	0.4317	Yes	C4	0.005	0.1	0.7383	0.1910
Yes	C5	0.008	0.2	0.6499	0.3647	Yes	C8	0.002	0.1	0.8070	0.8213
Yes	C9	0.038	1.0	0.3306	0.8501	Yes	C13	0.016	0.4	0.5282	0.5098
Yes	C16	0.014	0.3	0.5620	0.5937	No	C2	0.047	1.2	0.2863	0.4868
No	C3	0.152	4.3	0.0489	0.5339	No	C6	0.063	1.6	0.2169	0.9336
No	C7	0.088	2.3	0.1411	0.4787	No	C10	0.011	0.3	0.6176	0.4426
No	C11	0.003	0.1	0.7793	0.3594	No	C12	0.090	2.4	0.1360	0.4062
No	C14	0.012	0.3	0.5980	0.3687	No	C15	0.034	0.9	0.3655	0.4214
No	C17	0.135	3.7	0.0653	0.9233	No	C18	0.061	1.5	0.2256	0.4792
No	C19	0.005	0.1	0.7268	0.2016						

Overall Wilk's Lambda 0.7992

Classification Matrix

Classification Variable: C20
Independent Variables C1 C4 C5 C8 C9 C13 C16
Group Counts Table

	P(All)	P(1)	P(2)
A(All)	49	22	27
A(1)	22	12	10
A(2)	27	10	17

Percent reduction in classification error due to X's 18.4

Linear Discriminant Functions

Classification Variable: C20

Group	1	2
CONSTANT	−6.913793	−6.139007
C1	1.357363	1.125289
C4	0.3213706	0.2963162
C5	0.094547	0.084688
C8	0.1466019	0.1623168
C9	−0.1434003	−0.038856
C13	−0.007688	−0.012877
C16	0.0897661	0.098917

Misclassified Rows

Row	Act	Pred	P(1)	P(2)
2	1	2	0.492	0.508
3	1	2	0.349	0.651
5	1	2	0.361	0.639
11	1	2	0.380	0.620
13	1	2	0.129	0.871
18	1	2	0.249	0.751
20	1	2	0.362	0.638
21	1	2	0.000	1.000
24	1	2	0.441	0.559
25	1	2	0.290	0.710
32	2	1	0.773	0.227
36	2	1	0.706	0.294
39	2	1	0.504	0.496
40	2	1	0.536	0.464
41	2	1	0.587	0.413
43	2	1	0.576	0.424
46	2	1	0.510	0.490
48	2	1	0.535	0.465
50	2	1	0.627	0.373
52	2	1	0.596	0.404

Group Counts Report

Group	Count
All	32
1	12
2	20

Variable Selection Report

Classification Variable: C20

IN	Variable	R2-Ad	F-Val	F-Prob	R2-Xs	IN	Variable	R2-Ad	F-Val	F-Prob	R2-Xs
Yes	C1	0.015	0.4	0.5513	0.5590	Yes	C4	0.002	0.0	0.8427	0.1898
Yes	C5	0.033	0.8	0.3765	0.4675	Yes	C8	0.002	0.0	0.8306	0.8329
Yes	C9	0.007	0.2	0.6849	0.8775	Yes	C13	0.017	0.4	0.5214	0.5753
Yes	C16	0.006	0.1	0.7181	0.5873	No	C2	0.008	0.2	0.6727	0.4728
No	C3	0.129	3.4	0.0782	0.4054	No	C6	0.075	1.9	0.1851	0.4723
No	C7	0.007	0.2	0.6911	0.6218	No	C10	0.002	0.0	0.8388	0.5406
No	C11	0.020	0.5	0.5053	0.3922	No	C12	0.116	3.0	0.0951	0.2857
No	C14	0.027	0.6	0.4338	0.5907	No	C15	0.042	1.0	0.3238	0.3903
No	C17	0.115	3.0	0.0971	0.8324	No	C18	0.006	0.1	0.7084	0.4522
No	C19	0.001	0.0	0.8706	0.3319						

Overall Wilk's Lambda 0.8513

Classification Matrix

Classification Variable: C20
Independent Variables C1 C4 C5 C8 C9 C13 C16
Group Counts Table

	P(All)	P(1)	P(2)
A(All)	45	20	25
A(1)	22	12	10
A(2)	23	8	15

Percent reduction in classification error due to X's 20.0

Linear Discriminant Functions

Classification Variable: C20

Group	1	2
CONSTANT	−20.76216	−19.58388
C1	6.785572	6.438477
C4	0.6820685	0.6633766
C5	0.1996382	0.1793405
C8	0.2960492	0.2796331
C9	−0.3849141	−0.3283038
C13	−0.013707	−0.008446
C16	0.4984985	0.5134127

Misclassified Rows

Row	Act	Pred	P(1)	P(2)
2	1	2	0.231	0.769
3	1	2	0.227	0.773
7	1	2	0.377	0.623
10	1	2	0.315	0.685
11	1	2	0.474	0.526
13	1	2	0.241	0.759
16	1	2	0.257	0.743
18	1	2	0.335	0.665
20	1	2	0.109	0.891
23	1	2	0.043	0.957
36	2	1	0.595	0.405
37	2	1	0.521	0.479
38	2	1	0.579	0.421
39	2	1	0.565	0.435
40	2	1	0.550	0.450
42	2	1	0.714	0.286
44	2	1	0.711	0.289
48	2	1	0.711	0.289

Appendix C

Comparison of Values of Nineteen Variables Before Merger and One Year After Merger

Two Sample T-Test Results

	C1		C1	
Count – Mean	26	3.326154	21	2.607143
95% C.L. of Mean	1.975226	4.677082	2.024127	3.190159
Std. Dev. – Std. Error	3.344896	0.655988	1.280883	0.2795116
	---- Equal Variances ----		---- Unequal Variances ----	
T Value – Prob.	0.9299277	0.3574	1.008353	0.3204
Degrees of Freedom		45		34.22837
Diff. – Std. Error	0.7190108	0.7731901	0.7190108	0.7130547
95% C.L. of Diff.	−0.8382528	2.276274	−0.7300227	2.168044
F-ratio testing group variances		6.819401	Prob. Level	0.0000

```
      | .9                    95% Conf. Limit Plots                   18.69|
   C1 | <-----a----->                                                     |
   C1 |   <a->                                                            |
      | .9                        Line Plots                         18.69|
   C1 | .2146222.1121....1........................................1       |
   C1 | 11244212..2....11................................................ |
```

Two Sample T-Test Results

	C2		C2	
Count – Mean	20	1.621	16	0.900625
95% C.L. of Mean	0.3179529	2.924047	0.5269628	1.274287
Std. Dev. – Std. Error	2.784687	0.622675	0.7014791	0.1753698
	---- Equal Variances ----		---- Unequal Variances ----	
T Value – Prob.	1.006825	0.3211	1.113582	0.2775
Degrees of Freedom		34		22.27493
Diff. – Std. Error	0.7203751	0.715492	0.7203751	0.6468993
95% C.L. of Diff.	−0.7336702	2.17442	−0.6210697	2.06182
F-ratio testing group variances		15.75881	Prob. Level	0.0000

```
      .02          95% Conf. Limit Plots            13.1
C2   | <-----a----->                                    |
C2   |   <-a>                                           |
      .02               Line Plots                  13.1
C2   | 11434.22.1...1...........................................1|
C2   | 11533..1.1..1..........................................  |
```

Two Sample T-Test Results

	C3		C3	
Count – Mean	26	73.65769	21	81.76476
95% C.L. of Mean	64.19968	83.1157	71.68442	91.84511
Std. Dev. – Std. Error	23.41802	4.592651	22.14645	4.832751
	---- Equal Variances ----		---- Unequal Variances ----	
T Value – Prob.	−1.208661	0.2331	−1.216013	0.2302
Degrees of Freedom		45		45.86832
Diff. – Std. Error	−8.107071	6.70748	−8.107071	6.666927
95% C.L. of Diff.	−21.61645	5.402304	−21.52687	5.312731
F-ratio testing group variances		1.118129	Prob. Level	0.4037

```
   26.34             95% Conf. Limit Plots        123.57
C3 |                       <-----a---->                 |
C3 |                        <----a----->                |
   26.34                   Line Plots               123.57
C3 | 1.....1...1.11.2..2...1.1..11.1....1113121....1........1...|
C3 | ..........1....2..1...11.1111.....1...2.2.111...1.1......1|
```

Two Sample T-Test Results

	C4		C4	
Count – Mean	26	5.375769	21	5.594286
95% C.L. of Mean	3.866084	6.885455	4.30895	6.879621
Std. Dev. – Std. Error	3.737979	0.7330781	2.823874	0.6162199

	---- Equal Variances ----		---- Unequal Variances ----	
T Value – Prob.	−0.2214956	0.8257	−0.2281752	0.8205
Degrees of Freedom		45		46.75937
Diff. – Std. Error	−0.2185164	0.9865494	−0.2185164	0.9576693
95% C.L. of Diff.	−2.205502	1.768469	−2.145327	1.708295

F-ratio testing group variances		1.752198	Prob. Level	0.1020

```
     .65                    95% Conf. Limit Plots               17.86
C4   |              <----a---->                                     |
C4   |              <---a---->                                      |
     .65                         Line Plots                   17.86
C4   | 1....21131221..1112.112.1........................1.........1 |
C4   | ...1.11112....2111112.12........1..........1.............    |
```

Two Sample T-Test Results

	C5		C5	
Count – Mean	24	36.80333	20	36.458
95% C.L. of Mean	29.47025	44.13641	26.64999	46.26601
Std. Dev. – Std. Error	17.36787	3.545202	20.96029	4.686863

	---- Equal Variances ----		---- Unequal Variances ----	
T Value – Prob.	5.978918E-02	0.9526	5.876349E-02	0.9534
Degrees of Freedom		42		38.71051
Diff. – Std. Error	0.3453331	5.775847	0.3453331	5.876661
95% C.L. of Diff.	−11.31076	12.00143	−11.54381	12.23448

F-ratio testing group variances		1.456469	Prob. Level	0.1938

```
     5.42                   95% Conf. Limit Plots               70.06
C5   |              <------a----->                                  |
C5   |              <-------a-------->                               |
     5.42                        Line Plots                    70.06
C5   | ..1..11...11.1..11....1..11..111..21.1....1..3...1......1.    |
C5   | 1...1..11..2.2......1.......11...1..2..1.....1.1.....1..11     |
```

Two Sample T-Test Results

	C6		C6	
Count – Mean	25	9.0736	21	121.0114
95% C.L. of Mean	4.770141	13.37706	−123.5748	365.5977
Std. Dev. – Std. Error	10.42585	2.085171	537.3543	117.2603

	---- Equal Variances ----		---- Unequal Variances ----	
T-Value – Prob.	−1.043591	0.3024	−0.9544586	0.3512
Degrees of Freedom		44		20.01391
Diff. – Std. Error	−111.9378	107.2622	−111.9378	117.2789
95% C.L. of Diff.	−328.1106	104.2349	−356.5586	132.6829

F-ratio testing group variances		2656.429	Prob. Level	0.0000

```
     |  -123.5748            95% Conf. Limit Plots          2,466.15 |
  C6 |                    <----a---->                                |
  C6 |                    <---a---->                                 |
     |  -123.5748               Line Plots                  2,466.15 |
  C6 |  ...01.................................................       |
  C6 |  ...K................................................1        |
```

Two Sample T-Test Results

	C7		C7	
Count – Mean	26	19.02962	21	32.16095
95% C.L. of Mean	12.52218	25.53705	14.95074	49.37117
Std. Dev. – Std. Error	16.1124	3.159902	37.81073	8.250977

	---- Equal Variances ----		---- Unequal Variances ----	
T-Value – Prob.	−1.602923	0.1159	−1.486225	0.1492
Degrees of Freedom		45		26.42837
Diff. – Std. Error	−13.13134	8.19212	−13.13134	8.835361
95% C.L. of Diff.	−29.63089	3.368214	−31.29127	5.028597

F-ratio testing group variances		5.50693	Prob. Level	0.0000

```
     |  .59                  95% Conf. Limit Plots           140.64 |
  C7 |          <--a->                                               |
  C7 |              <------a------>                                  |
     |  .59                     Line Plots                   140.64 |
  C7 |  112243232..11...1..1.1....1................................  |
  C7 |  1124.1122.1........1...1.1.........1..........1...........1  |
```

Two Sample T-Test Results

	C8		C8	
Count – Mean	26	12.94462	21	8.253333
95% C.L. of Mean	8.13383	17.7554	3.750531	12.75614
Std. Dev. – Std. Error	11.9115	2.336037	9.892626	2.158748

	---- Equal Variances ----		---- Unequal Variances ----	
T-Value – Prob.	1.445743	0.1552	1.474891	0.1469
Degrees of Freedom		45		46.97319
Diff. – Std. Error	4.691282	3.244893	4.691282	3.180764
95% C.L. of Diff.	−1.84418	11.22674	−1.707606	11.09017

F-ratio testing group variances		1.449805	Prob. Level	0.2000

```
    -7.24              95% Conf. Limit Plots              47.81
C8 |                        <----a---->                        |
C8 |                   <----a---->                             |
    -7.24                  Line Plots                     47.81
C8 | ..1......22.132..3.11..11.2..1..1.1.1........1...........1
C8 | 1.1...1..11..431111.1.1.1...............1..1.............. 
```


Two Sample T-Test Results

	C9		C9	
Count – Mean	26	6.891154	21	2.898095
95% C.L. of Mean	3.472609	10.3097	−1.243108	7.039299
Std. Dev. – Std. Error	8.464315	1.659989	9.098197	1.985389

	---- Equal Variances ----		---- Unequal Variances ----	
T-Value – Prob.	1.555107	0.1269	1.54296	0.1302
Degrees of Freedom		45		43.423
Diff. – Std. Error	3.993059	2.567708	3.993059	2.587921
95% C.L. of Diff.	−1.178499	9.164617	−1.224484	9.210602

F-ratio testing group variances		1.155386	Prob. Level	0.3620

```
    -18.83             95% Conf. Limit Plots              32.06
C9 |                        <---a--->                         |
C9 |                   <---a---->                             |
    -18.83                 Line Plots                     32.06
C9 | ............1......12221.2..2.34..1.2.1..........1.......1
C9 | 1..........1...1.131..12.1321.1.............1...1........ 
```

Two Sample T-Test Results

	C10		C10	
Count – Mean	26	1.359615	21	1.139524
95% C.L. of Mean	1.17336	1.545871	1.006794	1.272254
Std. Dev. – Std. Error	0.4611679	9.044247E-02	0.2916072	6.363391E-02

	---- Equal Variances ----		---- Unequal Variances ----	
T-Value – Prob.	1.899603	0.0639	1.990241	0.0528
Degrees of Freedom		45		44.3949
Diff. – Std. Error	0.2200915	0.1158618	0.2200915	0.1105853
95% C.L. of Diff.	−1.326308E-02	0.453446	−2.775624E-03	0.4429585

F-ratio testing group variances		2.501046	Prob. Level	0.0201

```
     .53                    95% Conf. Limit Plots                    2.7
C10  |                        <----a---->                              |
C10  |                     <--a-->                                     |
     .53                         Line Plots                        2.7
C10  |1.....1.2..1.1.212.2.1.121.2...1..2..11..................1       |
C10  |...1..1.11121.31.22.......113............................        |
```

Two Sample T-Test Results

	C11		C11	
Count – Mean	26	116601	21	126419.9
95% C.L. of Mean	94223.1	138979	104659.5	148180.3
Std. Dev. – Std. Error	55407.75	10866.35	47807.44	10432.44

	---- Equal Variances ----		---- Unequal Variances ----	
T-Value – Prob.	−0.6415275	0.5244	−0.6518254	0.5177
Degrees of Freedom		45		46.81457
Diff. – Std. Error	−9818.867	15305.45	−9818.867	15063.65
95% C.L. of Diff.	−40645.21	21007.47	−40125.7	20487.97

F-ratio testing group variances		1.343229	Prob. Level	0.2524

```
     10652                  95% Conf. Limit Plots                 236452
C11  |                        <-----a---->                             |
C11  |                            <----a----->                         |
     10652                       Line Plots                       236452
C11  |1...1..1...1.1.2..1...21.111..112...1..1111.11...........1       |
C11  |.........111.....1....2.2.2...11.1..2..31...1............1       |
```

Two Sample T-Test Results

	C12		C12	
Count – Mean	26	17.98	21	18.19524
95% C.L. of Mean	17.64227	18.31773	17.82759	18.56289
Std. Dev. – Std. Error	0.8362296	0.1639981	0.8077229	0.1762596
	---- Equal Variances ----		---- Unequal Variances ----	
T-Value – Prob.	−0.890652	0.3779	−0.8940161	0.3760
Degrees of Freedom		45		45.54506
Diff. – Std. Error	−0.2152386	0.2416641	−0.2152386	0.2407547
95% C.L. of Diff.	−0.7019683	0.2714912	−0.6998498	0.2693727
F-ratio testing group variances		1.071831	Prob. Level	0.4421

```
       16.07              95% Conf. Limit Plots                    19.61
C12  |                        <-----a----->                            |
C12  |                          <-----a------->                        |
       16.07                   Line Plots                         19.61
C12  |  1........1.....11..2....111.1...2112111.1....11.2....11....     |
C12  |  ......1.........1....21.....111...1.1211.1.1...1.1..11....1     |
```


Two Sample T-Test Results

	C13		C13	
Count – Mean	26	13.50654	21	−0.702381
95% C.L. of Mean	5.309295	21.70378	−19.91931	18.51455
Std. Dev. – Std. Error	20.29637	3.980445	42.21948	9.213044
	---- Equal Variances ----		---- Unequal Variances ----	
T-Value – Prob.	1.515585	0.1366	1.415775	0.1679
Degrees of Freedom		45		28.12444
Diff. – Std. Error	14.20892	9.375206	14.20892	10.03614
95% C.L. of Diff.	−4.673458	33.0913	−6.347839	34.76568
F-ratio testing group variances		4.327021	Prob. Level	0.0004

```
      -177.78             95% Conf. Limit Plots                     62.7
C13  |                                       <-a->                        |
C13  |                                      <----a---->                   |
      -177.78                  Line Plots                             62.7
C13  |  .............................1...1.1.2341622.....11.1            |
C13  |  1...........................1..232521.31........                  |
```

Two Sample T-Test Results

	C14		C14	
Count – Mean	26	170.7362	21	135.2276
95% C.L. of Mean	132.5612	208.9111	114.055	156.4003
Std. Dev. – Std. Error	94.52123	18.53714	46.51619	10.15066
	---- Equal Variances ----		---- Unequal Variances ----	
T-Value – Prob.	1.572283	0.1229	1.680133	0.1009
Degrees of Freedom		45		39.08587
Diff. – Std. Error	35.50855	22.58407	35.50855	21.13437
95% C.L. of Diff.	−9.97749	80.99458	−7.23597	78.25306
F-ratio testing group variances		4.129053	Prob. Level	0.0010

```
      | 54.81                95% Conf. Limit Plots                   435.57 |
C14   |             <-------a-------->                                     |
C14   |        <-----a----->                                              |
      | 54.81                    Line Plots                        435.57 |
C14   | 1..3.12.1.131.11.1.3...1......1...1..11.1.................1        |
C14   | ...121211.21112..2.1...11..1...............................       |
```

Two Sample T-Test Results

	C15		C15	
Count – Mean	26	107.89	21	168.8276
95% C.L. of Mean	65.71613	150.0639	29.39617	308.2591
Std. Dev. – Std. Error	104.4225	20.47893	306.33	66.84668
	---- Equal Variances ----		---- Unequal Variances ----	
T-Value – Prob.	−0.9503517	0.3470	−0.8716174	0.3921
Degrees of Freedom		45		24.1358
Diff. – Std. Error	−60.93762	64.12113	−60.93762	69.91327
95% C.L. of Diff.	−190.0825	68.20721	−205.2141	83.33882
F-ratio testing group variances		8.605796	Prob. Level	0.0000

```
      | 0                    95% Conf. Limit Plots                 1379.59 |
C15   |      <a->                                                          |
C15   |   <-----a------->                                                  |
      | 0                        Line Plots                        1379.59 |
C15   | 36214211211.1......1...............................                |
C15   | 271.33.1..1..1.........1...............................1           |
```

Two Sample T-Test Results

	C16		C16	
Count – Mean	26	18.13346	21	18.30571
95% C.L. of Mean	15.05579	21.21114	15.32373	21.28769
Std. Dev. – Std. Error	7.620318	1.494467	6.551388	1.42963

	---- Equal Variances ----		---- Unequal Variances ----	
T-Value – Prob.	−8.194076E-02	0.9351	−8.328798E-02	0.9340
Degrees of Freedom		45		46.83561
Diff. – Std. Error	−0.1722527	2.102161	−0.1722527	2.068157
95% C.L. of Diff.	−4.406165	4.061659	−4.33317	3.988665

F-ratio testing group variances		1.352943	Prob. Level	0.2471

```
     | 1.92              95% Conf. Limit Plots                 39.94|
C16  |                     <-----a------>                           |
C16  |                     <------a----->                           |
     | 1.92                    Line Plots                      39.94|
C16  | 1..........11111..122.1212..1...31.1..1.1................1    |
C16  | ..........1.1.21.3.....121.11.2..1.12...........1.........    |
```

Two Sample T-Test Results

	C17		C17	
Count – Mean	26	22.66308	21	21.48619
95% C.L. of Mean	15.92029	29.40586	14.51202	28.46036
Std. Dev. – Std. Error	16.69512	3.274183	15.3222	3.343579

	---- Equal Variances ----		---- Unequal Variances ----	
T-Value – Prob.	0.2491564	0.8044	0.2514862	0.8026
Degrees of Freedom		45		46.26203
Diff. – Std. Error	1.176886	4.723482	1.176886	4.679721
95% C.L. of Diff.	−8.336565	10.69034	−8.242829	10.5966

F-ratio testing group variances		1.187235	Prob. Level	0.3510

```
     | -12.94            95% Conf. Limit Plots                69.13|
C17  |                     <------a----->                           |
C17  |                     <------a----->                           |
     | -12.94                  Line Plots                      69.13|
C17  | .1......1..1.1..1.3.12211...212..1.1..111...............1    |
C17  | 1......1.........2.21..133121....1....1................1..    |
```

Appendix D

Comparison of Values of Nineteen Variables Before Merger and Two Years After Merger

Two Sample T-Test Results

	C1		C1	
Count – Mean	26	3.326154	15	2.493333
95% C.L. of Mean	1.975226	4.677082	1.836005	3.150661
Std. Dev. – Std. Error	3.344896	0.655988	1.187246	0.3065455

	---- Equal Variances ----		---- Unequal Variances ----	
T-Value – Prob.	0.9269743	0.3596	1.150179	0.2579
Degrees of Freedom		39		35.09461
Diff. – Std. Error	0.8328204	0.8984288	0.8328204	0.7240791
95% C.L. of Diff.	−0.9843853	2.650026	−0.6369605	2.302601

F-ratio testing group variances		7.937503	Prob. Level	0.0001

```
      | .9              95% Conf. Limit Plots            18.69|
C1    |         <-----a----->                                |
C1    |           <-a>                                       |
      | .9                   Line Plots                 18.69|
C1    | .2146222.1121....1.......................................1|
C1    | 21.33.1111.1.1...........................................|
```

Two Sample T-Test Results

	C2		C2	
Count – Mean	20	1.621	12	0.8458334
95% C.L. of Mean	0.3179529	2.924047	0.2513196	1.440347
Std. Dev. – Std. Error	2.784687	0.622675	0.9364969	0.2703434
	---- Equal Variances ----		---- Unequal Variances ----	
T-Value – Prob.	0.9280273	0.3608	1.141916	0.2639
Degrees of Freedom		30		26.05295
Diff. – Std. Error	0.7751667	0.8352844	0.7751667	0.6788297
95% C.L. of Diff.	−0.9306925	2.481026	−0.6201211	2.170455
F-ratio testing group variances		8.841789	Prob. Level	0.0004

```
        .04              95% Conf. Limit Plots                      13.1
C2   |   <-------a------->
C2   |   <---a-->
        .04                   Line Plots                           13.1
C2   |   11434.22.1..1..............................................1
C2   |   323..1.1...2..............................................
```


Two Sample T-Test Results

	C3		C3	
Count – Mean	26	73.65769	15	79.092
95% C.L. of Mean	64.19968	83.1157	66.51862	91.66539
Std. Dev. – Std. Error	23.41802	4.592651	22.70967	5.863612
	---- Equal Variances ----		---- Unequal Variances ----	
T-Value – Prob.	−0.7234849	0.4737	−0.7296225	0.4709
Degrees of Freedom		39		32.05725
Diff. – Std. Error	−5.434311	7.511299	−5.434311	7.448113
95% C.L. of Diff.	−20.62703	9.758407	−20.60531	9.736686
F-ratio testing group variances		1.063355	Prob. Level	0.4668

```
        26.34            95% Conf. Limit Plots                       118
C3   |                      <------a------->
C3   |                      <---------a--------->
        26.34                  Line Plots                            118
C3   |   1......1...1.11.2..2....11...2..1....111132.1....1........1
C3   |   ............2....1..1.1.11........2...1..1....11..1....1.
```

Two Sample T-Test Results

	C4		C4	
Count – Mean	26	5.375769	15	4.62
95% C.L. of Mean	3.866084	6.885455	3.257695	5.982305
Std. Dev. – Std. Error	3.737979	0.7330781	2.460555	0.6353124

	---- Equal Variances ----		---- Unequal Variances ----	
T-Value – Prob.	0.6986837	0.4889	0.7790917	0.4405
Degrees of Freedom		39		40.41383
Diff. – Std. Error	0.7557693	1.081705	0.7557693	0.9700646
95% C.L. of Diff.	−1.432139	2.943677	−1.204734	2.716273

F-ratio testing group variances		2.307851	Prob. Level	0.0528

```
      |.65                95% Conf. Limit Plots                    17.86|
  C4  |              <----a---->                                        |
  C4  |              <---a---->                                         |
      |.65                     Line Plots                        17.86|
  C4  |1....21131221..1112.112.1........................1.........1|
  C4  |2....11..1.1.12.21......2...1................................|
```

Two Sample T-Test Results

	C5		C5	
Count – Mean	24	36.80333	15	37.71
95% C.L. of Mean	29.47025	44.13641	24.59291	50.82708
Std. Dev. – Std. Error	17.36787	3.545202	23.69168	6.117165

	---- Equal Variances ----		---- Unequal Variances ----	
T-Value – Prob.	−0.1377514	0.8912	−0.1282371	0.8990
Degrees of Freedom		37		24.63038
Diff. – Std. Error	−0.9066658	6.581901	−0.9066658	7.070231
95% C.L. of Diff.	−14.24254	12.4292	−15.47744	13.66411

F-ratio testing group variances		1.860795	Prob. Level	0.0902

```
      |3.89               95% Conf. Limit Plots                   79.34|
  C5  |              <--------a------>                                  |
  C5  |              <---------a---------->                             |
      |3.89                    Line Plots                        79.34|
  C5  |...1.11...111..11...1..11.2.1.12.1...1.12..1.....1........|
  C5  |11.......11.1.....1...1....1.2..1..1............1.....1.1|
```

Two Sample T-Test Results

	C6		C6	
Count – Mean	25	9.0736	15	9.513333
95% C.L. of Mean	4.770141	13.37706	−4.054499	23.08117
Std. Dev. – Std. Error	10.42585	2.085171	24.50581	6.327373
	---- Equal Variances ----		---- Unequal Variances ----	
T-Value – Prob.	−0.079077	0.9374	−6.600524E-02	0.9481
Degrees of Freedom		38		17.52227
Diff. – Std. Error	−0.4397335	5.560827	−0.4397335	6.6621
95% C.L. of Diff.	−11.69699	10.81752	−14.43962	13.56015
F-ratio testing group variances		5.524778	Prob. Level	0.0001

```
    |  -4.054499           95% Conf. Limit Plots              97.13 |
C6  |      <---a---->                                               |
C6  |   <---------a--------->                                       |
    |  -4.054499               Line Plots                    97.13 |
C6  |  ...474111.3.....11..1...1..................................  |
C6  |  ..35211.11.................................................1 |
```

Two Sample T-Test Results

	C7		C7	
Count – Mean	26	19.02962	15	18.49333
95% C.L. of Mean	12.52218	25.53705	11.39894	25.58772
Std. Dev. – Std. Error	16.1124	3.159902	12.81367	3.308476
	---- Equal Variances ----		---- Unequal Variances ----	
T-Value – Prob.	0.1101789	0.9128	0.117219	0.9073
Degrees of Freedom		39		37.18299
Diff. – Std. Error	0.5362816	4.867373	0.5362816	4.57504
95% C.L. of Diff.	−9.308703	10.38127	−8.731928	9.804491
F-ratio testing group variances		1.58115	Prob. Level	0.1869

```
    |  .59                 95% Conf. Limit Plots              65.19 |
C7  |          <------a------->                                     |
C7  |          <-------a------->                                    |
    |  .59                     Line Plots                    65.19 |
C7  |  1.1.2.1131211.12111.....1.1........1.....1....1..........1   |
C7  |  .1.11.1...2..111.1.1..1.......1...1....1.................:.  |
```

Two Sample T-Test Results

	C8		C8	
Count – Mean	26	12.94462	15	8.741333
95% C.L. of Mean	8.13383	17.7554	2.45435	15.02832
Std. Dev. – Std. Error	11.9115	2.336037	11.35536	2.931941

	---- Equal Variances ----		---- Unequal Variances ----	
T-Value – Prob.	1.106599	0.2752	1.12124	0.2703
Degrees of Freedom		39		32.51864
Diff. – Std. Error	4.203282	3.798377	4.203282	3.748779
95% C.L. of Diff.	−3.4795	11.88606	−3.427501	11.83407

F-ratio testing group variances	1.100351	Prob. Level	0.4387

```
    |-8.38                95% Conf. Limit Plots              47.81|
C8  |                     <------a------>                         |
C8  |                  <---------a------>                         |
    |-8.38                   Line Plots                     47.81|
C8  |....1.....22.132..3.11..1111..1.1..11........1...........1   |
C8  |1.1.......2.2.112.....1...1..1.........11..................  |
```


Two Sample T-Test Results

	C9		C9	
Count – Mean	26	6.891154	15	3.278
95% C.L. of Mean	3.472609	10.3097	−2.307045	8.863046
Std. Dev. – Std. Error	8.464315	1.659989	10.08754	2.604591

	---- Equal Variances ----		---- Unequal Variances ----	
T-Value – Prob.	1.227211	0.2271	1.169835	0.2523
Degrees of Freedom		39		26.82017
Diff. – Std. Error	3.613154	2.944201	3.613154	3.088601
95% C.L. of Diff.	−2.341929	9.568236	−2.725628	9.951935

F-ratio testing group variances	1.420322	Prob. Level	0.2152

```
    |-16.88               95% Conf. Limit Plots              32.06|
C9  |                       <-----a----->                         |
C9  |                   <-------a-------->                         |
    |-16.88                   Line Plots                     32.06|
C9  |..........1.......2141..2.11124..1.2.1............1.......1   |
C9  |1.....1....1.....1.....312.1..1...1......1..1............     |
```

Two Sample T-Test Results

	C10		C10	
Count – Mean	26	1.359615	15	1.201333
95% C.L. of Mean	1.17336	1.545871	1.048745	1.353921
Std. Dev. – Std. Error	0.4611679	9.044247E-02	0.2755998	7.115956E-02

	---- Equal Variances ----		---- Unequal Variances ----	
T-Value – Prob.	1.206938	0.2347	1.375403	0.1756
Degrees of Freedom		39		40.98064
Diff. – Std. Error	0.158282	0.1311435	0.158282	0.1150805
95% C.L. of Diff.	−0.1069752	0.4235393	−0.0741268	0.3906909

F-ratio testing group variances		2.800015	Prob. Level	0.0242

```
      |.53               95% Conf. Limit Plots                2.7|
C10   |                     <------a------>                      |
C10   |                     <-----a----->                       |
      |.53                      Line Plots                   2.7|
C10   |1.....1.2..1.1.212.2.1.121.2...1..2..11..................1|
C10   |.......111.2.1..1..1..21.211.............................|
```


Two Sample T-Test Results

	C11		C11	
Count – Mean	26	116601	15	126184.2
95% C.L. of Mean	94223.1	138979	106425.3	145943.1
Std. Dev. – Std. Error	55407.75	10866.35	35687.87	9214.568

	---- Equal Variances ----		---- Unequal Variances ----	
T-Value – Prob.	−0.6001768	0.5519	−0.6726296	0.5050
Degrees of Freedom		39		40.61067
Diff. – Std. Error	−9583.164	15967.24	−9583.164	14247.31
95% C.L. of Diff.	−41879.27	22712.94	−38363.72	19197.39

F-ratio testing group variances		2.41046	Prob. Level	0.0445

```
      |10652             95% Conf. Limit Plots             234563|
C11   |                     <-------a------->                    |
C11   |                     <------a------>                      |
      |10652                    Line Plots                 234563|
C11   |1...1..1...1.1.2..1...21.111..1111..1...21.111..........1 |
C11   |..........2...........111.11.1.11.1.31....................|
```

Two Sample T-Test Results

	C12		C12	
Count – Mean	26	17.98	15	18.11067
95% C.L. of Mean	17.64227	18.31773	17.63141	18.58993
Std. Dev. – Std. Error	0.8362296	0.1639981	0.865625	0.2235034

	---- Equal Variances ----		---- Unequal Variances ----	
T-Value – Prob.	−0.4758539	0.6368	−0.4713521	0.6408
Degrees of Freedom		39		30.31582
Diff. – Std. Error	−0.1306667	0.2745942	−0.1306667	0.2772168
95% C.L. of Diff.	−0.6860743	0.4247409	−0.6967545	0.4354211

F-ratio testing group variances		1.07154	Prob. Level	0.4248

```
       16.07              95% Conf. Limit Plots                  19.36
C12 |                            <-----a----->                        |
C12 |                            <-------a--------->                   |
       16.07                   Line Plots                        19.36
C12 | 1.......1......11..2.....2.1.1...12112.11.1....1.111....11|
C12 | ....1...1..............1..1.....1.12...11.1.1....1.1....1|
```

Two Sample T-Test Results

	C13		C13	
Count – Mean	26	13.50654	15	−61.192
95% C.L. of Mean	5.309295	21.70378	−186.5604	64.17641
Std. Dev. – Std. Error	20.29637	3.980445	226.4366	58.46569

	---- Equal Variances ----		---- Unequal Variances ----	
T-Value – Prob.	1.68609	0.0998	1.274697	0.2232
Degrees of Freedom		39		14.14846
Diff. – Std. Error	74.69854	44.30281	74.69854	58.60103
95% C.L. of Diff.	−14.91048	164.3076	−50.94283	200.3399

F-ratio testing group variances		124.4677	Prob. Level	0.0000

```
     -856.01              95% Conf. Limit Plots               64.17641
C13 |                                                           <a    |
C13 |                                  <----------a---------->        |
     -856.01                   Line Plots                     64.17641
C13 | ....................................................116D221|
C13 | 1..........................................1..........2362..|
```

Two Sample T-Test Results

	C14		C14	
Count – Mean	26	170.7362	15	148.9187
95% C.L. of Mean	132.5612	208.9111	117.3102	180.5272
Std. Dev. – Std. Error	94.52123	18.53714	57.09032	14.74066

	---- Equal Variances ----		---- Unequal Variances ----	
T-Value – Prob.	0.8102368	0.4227	0.921207	0.3623
Degrees of Freedom		39		40.95703
Diff. – Std. Error	21.81749	26.9273	21.81749	23.68359
95% C.L. of Diff.	−32.64698	76.28195	−26.0131	69.64807

F-ratio testing group variances		2.741155	Prob. Level	0.0264

```
        | 54.81              95% Conf. Limit Plots              435.57 |
    C14 |              <----a---->                                     |
    C14 |              <---a---->                                      |
        | 54.81                   Line Plots                     435.57 |
    C14 | 1..3.12.1.131.11.1.3...1......1...1..11.1.................1   |
    C14 | ....11112..1.1111....1.1.....1.1..........................   |
```


Two Sample T-Test Results

	C15		C15	
Count – Mean	26	107.89	15	476.45
95% C.L. of Mean	65.71613	150.0639	−216.1866	1169.087
Std. Dev. – Std. Error	104.4225	20.47893	1251.019	323.0118

	---- Equal Variances ----		---- Unequal Variances ----	
T-Value – Prob.	−1.50719	0.1398	−1.138725	0.2739
Degrees of Freedom		39		14.12873
Diff. – Std. Error	−368.56	244.5346	−368.56	323.6603
95% C.L. of Diff.	−863.1676	126.0476	−1062.516	325.3956

F-ratio testing group variances		143.5291	Prob. Level	0.0000

```
        | -216.1866           95% Conf. Limit Plots            4864.95 |
    C15 |    <a                                                        |
    C15 | <-------a--------->                                          |
        | -216.1866                Line Plots                   4864.95 |
    C15 | ..2D6311.................................................    |
    C15 | ..174.1.........1....................................1       |
```

Two Sample T-Test Results

	C16		C16	
Count – Mean	26	18.13346	15	19.806
95% C.L. of Mean	15.05579	21.21114	14.36315	25.24885
Std. Dev. – Std. Error	7.620318	1.494467	9.830707	2.538278
	---- Equal Variances ----		---- Unequal Variances ----	
T-Value – Prob.	−0.6082797	0.5465	−0.5678182	0.5752
Degrees of Freedom		39		25.08671
Diff. – Std. Error	−1.672539	2.749621	−1.672539	2.945554
95% C.L. of Diff.	−7.234057	3.888979	−7.737543	4.392465
F-ratio testing group variances		1.664268	Prob. Level	0.1293

```
     | 1.92            95% Conf. Limit Plots          39.94|
 C16 |                    <-----a------>                   |
 C16 |                  <---------a----------->            |
     | 1.92                 Line Plots                39.94|
 C16 | 1.........11111..122.1212..1...31.1..1.1.............1|
 C16 | ..........1.2.11111.....11............1..1..1.1.......1..|
```


Two Sample T-Test Results

	C17		C17	
Count – Mean	26	22.66308	15	18.77867
95% C.L. of Mean	15.92029	29.40586	9.060896	28.49644
Std. Dev. – Std. Error	16.69512	3.274183	17.55194	4.531893
	---- Equal Variances ----		---- Unequal Variances ----	
T-Value – Prob.	0.704402	0.4854	0.6947717	0.4925
Degrees of Freedom		39		29.91029
Diff. – Std. Error	3.884409	5.514478	3.884409	5.590914
95% C.L. of Diff.	−7.269442	15.03826	−7.533929	15.30275
F-ratio testing group variances		1.105277	Prob. Level	0.3994

```
     | -11.79          95% Conf. Limit Plots          69.13|
 C17 |                    <---a---->                       |
 C17 |                  <------a----->                     |
     | -11.79               Line Plots                69.13|
 C17 | 1.......1.1..1..121.2311...1121..11..1.2................1|
 C17 | ......111...11.1..1.1....211....1.......1.......1.........|
```

Two Sample T-Test Results

	C18		C18	
Count – Mean	26	5.507692	15	5.833334
95% C.L. of Mean	5.096622	5.918763	5.321316	6.345351
Std. Dev. – Std. Error	1.017811	0.1996091	0.9247909	.23878

	---- Equal Variances ----		---- Unequal Variances ----	
T-Value – Prob.	−1.019187	0.3144	−1.046328	0.3028
Degrees of Freedom		39		33.81207
Diff. – Std. Error	−0.3256412	0.3195106	−0.3256412	0.3112229
95% C.L. of Diff.	−0.9718989	0.3206165	−0.9581375	0.3068552

F-ratio testing group variances		1.211287	Prob. Level	0.3624

```
     |  3.3              95% Conf. Limit Plots                8.3|
C18  |                        <----a---->                         |
C18  |                       <-----a----->                        |
     |  3.3                    Line Plots                    8.3|
C18  |  1........11..1.11..2..3.1123..111.1.1........1.1....1......|
C18  |  ..............111.....11.11..23....1...1...............1|
```

Two Sample T-Test Results

	C19		C19	
Count – Mean	26	62	15	63.1
95% C.L. of Mean	55.18938	68.81062	57.55793	68.64208
Std. Dev. – Std. Error	16.8631	3.307125	10.00992	2.584551

	---- Equal Variances ----		---- Unequal Variances ----	
T-Value – Prob.	−0.2296424	0.8196	−0.2620754	0.7946
Degrees of Freedom		39		40.99077
Diff. – Std. Error	−1.099998	4.790051	−1.099998	4.197259
95% C.L. of Diff.	−10.78859	8.588591	−9.576437	7.37644

F-ratio testing group variances		2.838004	Prob. Level	0.0228

```
     |  18.8             95% Conf. Limit Plots               91.1|
C19  |                      <------a-------->                      |
C19  |                        <---a--->                           |
     |  18.8                   Line Plots                    91.1|
C19  |  1...1...........1....1..1.1..1111..1221..3211...1.....1..1|
C19  |  ...............1..1.....1.....1..12111211..1............|
```

Appendix E

Comparison of Values of Nineteen Variables Before Merger and Three Years After Merger

Two Sample T-Test Results

	C1		C1	
Count – Mean	26	3.326154	16	2.476875
95% C.L. of Mean	1.975226	4.677082	1.843773	3.109977
Std. Dev. – Std. Error	3.344896	0.655988	1.188527	0.2971317

	---- Equal Variances ----		---- Unequal Variances ----	
T-Value – Prob.	0.9745255	0.3357	1.179318	0.2462
Degrees of Freedom		40		34.75808
Diff. – Std. Error	0.8492787	0.871492	0.8492787	0.7201442
95% C.L. of Diff.	−0.9120398	2.610597	−0.6129977	2.311555

F-ratio testing group variances		7.920402	Prob. Level	0.0001

```
      1.15                95% Conf. Limit Plots                 18.69
C1  |      <-----a----->                                             |
C1  |    <---a--->                                                   |
      1.15                    Line Plots                       18.69 |
C1  | 2126233.1112....1.........................................1    |
C1  | .343.1.21..1..1................................................|
```

Two Sample T-Test Results

	C2		C2	
Count – Mean	20	1.621	12	0.9978333
95% C.L. of Mean	0.3179529	2.924047	0.364352	1.631315
Std. Dev. – Std. Error	2.784687	0.622675	0.9978797	0.2880631

	---- Equal Variances ----		---- Unequal Variances ----	
T-Value – Prob.	0.742969	0.4633	0.9083016	0.3718
Degrees of Freedom		30		26.81837
Diff. – Std. Error	0.6231667	0.838752	0.6231667	0.6860791
95% C.L. of Diff.	−1.089774	2.336108	−0.7848877	2.031221

F-ratio testing group variances		7.787471	Prob. Level	0.0006

```
       |.046              95% Conf. Limit Plots              13.1|
    C2 |  <-------a-------->                                     |
    C2 |  <----a---->                                            |
       |.046                  Line Plots                     13.1|
    C2 |11434.22.1..1...........................................1|
    C2 |22211..12.....1.........................................|
```

Two Sample T-Test Results

	C3		C3	
Count – Mean	26	73.65769	16	76.20937
95% C.L. of Mean	64.19968	83.1157	65.23543	87.18332
Std. Dev. – Std. Error	23.41802	4.592651	20.60147	5.150368

	---- Equal Variances ----		---- Unequal Variances ----	
T-Value – Prob.	−0.3584558	0.7219	−0.369775	0.7137
Degrees of Freedom		40		37.18457
Diff. – Std. Error	−2.551682	7.118539	−2.551682	6.900633
95% C.L. of Diff.	−16.93873	11.83537	−16.53111	11.42774

F-ratio testing group variances		1.292123	Prob. Level	0.3076

```
       |26.34             95% Conf. Limit Plots              118|
    C3 |                    <------a-------->                    |
    C3 |                    <--------a--------->                 |
       |26.34                 Line Plots                     118|
    C3 |1......1...1.11.2..2....11...2..1....111132.1....1.......1|
    C3 |......1.......1....1..2..1...11...2.2...1........12.......|
```

Two Sample T-Test Results

	C4		C4	
Count – Mean	26	5.375769	16	5.645
95% C.L. of Mean	3.866084	6.885455	4.230235	7.059765
Std. Dev. – Std. Error	3.737979	0.7330781	2.655949	0.6639873

	---- Equal Variances ----		---- Unequal Variances ----	
T-Value – Prob.	−0.2511958	0.8029	−0.2722029	0.7868
Degrees of Freedom		40		41.24578
Diff. – Std. Error	−0.2692308	1.071797	−0.2692308	0.9890817
95% C.L. of Diff.	−2.435405	1.896943	−2.266338	1.727877

F-ratio testing group variances		1.980771	Prob. Level	0.0853

```
     .65                   95% Conf. Limit Plots                    17.86
C4   |              <------a------>                                      |
C4   |            <------a----->                                        |
     .65                      Line Plots                             17.86
C4   |1....21131221..1112.112.1.........................1.........1      |
C4   |..2....1...1.211.1..1.21..1.1..1..............................     |
```

Two Sample T-Test Results

	C5		C5	
Count – Mean	24	36.80333	15	37.44867
95% C.L. of Mean	29.47025	44.13641	27.02316	47.87417
Std. Dev. – Std. Error	17.36787	3.545202	18.83024	4.861946

	---- Equal Variances ----		---- Unequal Variances ----	
T-Value – Prob.	−0.1093189	0.9135	−0.1072475	0.9153
Degrees of Freedom		37		29.78637
Diff. – Std. Error	−0.6453323	5.903206	−0.6453323	6.017223
95% C.L. of Diff.	−12.60607	11.31541	−12.93476	11.6441

F-ratio testing group variances		1.175488	Prob. Level	0.3543

```
     4.4                  95% Conf. Limit Plots                     69.08
C5   |              <--------a--------->                                 |
C5   |           <----------a----------->                               |
     4.4                     Line Plots                             69.08
C5   |...1..11...11.1..11...1...11..2.1..21.1....1.12...1......1         |
C5   |1.......1.2.........1.........11..11.11.1....1......1.....1        |
```

Two Sample T-Test Results

	C6		C6	
Count – Mean	25	9.0736	16	3.651875
95% C.L. of Mean	4.770141	13.37706	2.304493	4.999257
Std. Dev. – Std. Error	10.42585	2.085171	2.529451	0.6323628

	---- Equal Variances ----		---- Unequal Variances ----	
T-Value – Prob.	2.033507	0.0488	2.488229	0.0188
Degrees of Freedom		39		28.60645
Diff. – Std. Error	5.421725	2.666195	5.421725	2.178949
95% C.L. of Diff.	2.894926E-02	10.8145	0.9629631	9.880487

F-ratio testing group variances	16.98911	Prob. Level	0.0000

```
     |.56                95% Conf. Limit Plots               39.23|
C6   |      <--------a------->                                    |
C6   |   <---a--->                                                |
     |.56                    Line Plots                     39.23|
C6   |13231221..2..1....1.2..............1.1........1.........1   |
C6   |1232122..11...1............................................ |
```

Two Sample T-Test Results

	C7		C7	
Count – Mean	26	19.02962	16	23.685
95% C.L. of Mean	12.52218	25.53705	11.57571	35.79429
Std. Dev. – Std. Error	16.1124	3.159902	22.73286	5.683215

	---- Equal Variances ----		---- Unequal Variances ----	
T-Value – Prob.	−0.7764658	0.4420	−0.7159256	0.4807
Degrees of Freedom		40		25.48186
Diff. – Std. Error	−4.655384	5.995607	−4.655384	6.502608
95% C.L. of Diff.	−16.77291	7.462143	−18.03455	8.723782

F-ratio testing group variances	1.990617	Prob. Level	0.0619

```
     |-2.65              95% Conf. Limit Plots              70.62|
C7   |         <------a--------->                                |
C7   |         <----------a------------->                        |
     |-2.65                  Line Plots                    70.62|
C7   |...11.2.123121.1212.....1.1......1.....1...1.........1.... |
C7   |1.1...1.13.1..1..1.........1......1...11.........1.......1 |
```

Two Sample T-Test Results

	C8		C8	
Count – Mean	26	12.94462	16	8.880625
95% C.L. of Mean	8.13383	17.7554	3.480843	14.28041
Std. Dev. – Std. Error	11.9115	2.336037	10.13705	2.534263
	---- Equal Variances ----		---- Unequal Variances ----	
T-Value – Prob.	1.133992	0.2635	1.179105	0.2457
Degrees of Freedom		40		37.98611
Diff. – Std. Error	4.063991	3.58379	4.063991	3.446674
95% C.L. of Diff.	−3.179092	11.30707	−2.913416	11.0414
F-ratio testing group variances		1.380732	Prob. Level	0.2610

```
      -4.88                95% Conf. Limit Plots              47.81
C8   |               <--------a-------->                          |
C8   |          <-----a----->                                    |
      -4.88                    Line Plots                    47.81
C8   | 1......22.123..121.1..1111..1.1..1.1........1............1 |
C8   | ......11.2122221.................1.............1........ |
```

Two Sample T-Test Results

	C9		C9	
Count – Mean	26	6.891154	16	2.916875
95% C.L. of Mean	3.472609	10.3097	−1.251418	7.085168
Std. Dev. – Std. Error	8.464315	1.659989	7.825171	1.956293
	---- Equal Variances ----		---- Unequal Variances ----	
T-Value – Prob.	1.519695	0.1365	1.549024	0.1301
Degrees of Freedom		40		35.91707
Diff. – Std. Error	3.974279	2.615181	3.974279	2.565666
95% C.L. of Diff.	−1.311179	9.259737	−1.229172	9.17773
F-ratio testing group variances		1.420322	Prob. Level	0.3842

```
      -14.26               95% Conf. Limit Plots              32.06
C9   |                <-----a----->                             |
C9   |            <-----a----->                                 |
      -14.26                   Line Plots                    32.06
C9   | ........1.......2141..2..2.223..111.1...........1........1 |
C9   | 1............1...422.121...........1.........1.......... |
```

Two Sample T-Test Results

	C10		C10	
Count – Mean	26	1.359615	16	1.14
95% C.L. of Mean	1.17336	1.545871	0.9863892	1.293611
Std. Dev. – Std. Error	0.4611679	9.044247E-02	0.2883748	7.209369E-02

	---- Equal Variances ----		---- Unequal Variances ----	
T-Value – Prob.	1.706163	0.0957	1.898794	0.0645
Degrees of Freedom		40		41.99913
Diff. – Std. Error	0.2196153	0.1287188	0.2196153	0.1156605
95% C.L. of Diff.	−4.053411E-02	0.4797648	−1.379593E-02	0.4530266

F-ratio testing group variances		2.55743	Prob. Level	0.0311

```
     |.51                   95% Conf. Limit Plots                       2.7|
C10  |                    <-------a------->                              |
C10  |               <-------a------->                                  |
     |.51                       Line Plots                             2.7|
C10  |.1.....1.2.1.1.113.11.1.3.111..1..2..11...................1        |
C10  |1........113.112.1..11.1...1.1...........................        |
```

Two Sample T-Test Results

	C11		C11	
Count – Mean	26	116601	16	138855.4
95% C.L. of Mean	94223.1	138979	115895.2	161815.5
Std. Dev. – Std. Error	55407.75	10866.35	43103.31	10775.83

	---- Equal Variances ----		---- Unequal Variances ----	
T-Value – Prob.	−1.369499	0.1785	−1.454202	0.1537
Degrees of Freedom		40		39.88361
Diff. – Std. Error	−22254.34	16249.99	−22254.34	15303.47
95% C.L. of Diff.	−55096.66	10587.99	−53183.94	8675.264

F-ratio testing group variances		1.652417	Prob. Level	0.1567

```
     |10652                 95% Conf. Limit Plots                   234563|
C11  |                    <------a-------->                             |
C11  |                      <--------a------->                          |
     |10652                     Line Plots                          234563|
C11  |1...1..1...1.1.2..1...21.111..1111..1...21.111...........1        |
C11  |...........1...1......1..1.2.1.11.1.11..11..1.........1..         |
```

Two Sample T-Test Results

	C12		C12	
Count – Mean	26	17.98	16	18.25063
95% C.L. of Mean	17.64227	18.31773	17.83364	18.66761
Std. Dev. – Std. Error	0.8362296	0.1639981	0.7828109	0.1957027
	---- Equal Variances ----		---- Unequal Variances ----	
T-Value – Prob.	−1.042986	0.3032	−1.059895	0.2963
Degrees of Freedom		40		35.58843
Diff. – Std. Error	−0.2706261	0.2594724	−0.2706261	0.255333
95% C.L. of Diff.	−0.7950373	0.2537852	−0.7884852	0.2472331
F-ratio testing group variances		1.141136	Prob. Level	0.4045

```
      16.07            95% Conf. Limit Plots                   19.53
C12 |                                                              |
C12 |            <------a----------->                              |
    |                <--------a----------->                        |
      16.07                Line Plots                       19.53
C12 | 1.......1......2..2.....2.1.1..11121111.1....11.2....11...    |
C12 | ....1.................1..1...11...1.1.1...211.11...1......1    |
```


Two Sample T-Test Results

	C13		C13	
Count – Mean	26	13.50654	16	10.91
95% C.L. of Mean	5.309295	21.70378	3.758004	18.062
Std. Dev. – Std. Error	20.29637	3.980445	13.4265	3.356625
	---- Equal Variances ----		---- Unequal Variances ----	
T-Value – Prob.	0.4532431	0.6528	0.4986812	0.6206
Degrees of Freedom		40		41.84208
Diff. – Std. Error	2.596539	5.728798	2.596539	5.206811
95% C.L. of Diff.	−8.981751	14.17483	−7.911262	13.10434
F-ratio testing group variances		2.28513	Prob. Level	0.0495

```
     -35.67            95% Conf. Limit Plots                   62.7
C13 |                                                              |
C13 |           <---a-------->                                     |
    |              <-----a------->                                 |
     -35.67               Line Plots                        62.7
C13 | 1..........1.....1...212.13..341..12..............1.1....1   |
C13 | ............1.....1.23222.....1....1...........1.......      |
```

Two Sample T-Test Results

	C14		C14	
Count – Mean	26	170.7362	16	144.9144
95% C.L. of Mean	132.5612	208.9111	111.1627	178.6661
Std. Dev. – Std. Error	94.52123	18.53714	63.36234	15.84059

	---- Equal Variances ----		---- Unequal Variances ----	
T-Value – Prob.	0.9651657	0.3403	1.058991	0.2957
Degrees of Freedom		40		41.76504
Diff. – Std. Error	25.82179	26.75374	25.82179	24.38339
95% C.L. of Diff.	−28.24932	79.89291	−23.38614	75.02972

F-ratio testing group variances		2.225339	Prob. Level	0.0550

```
      | 54.81                   95% Conf. Limit Plots                   435.57 |
  C14 |               <--------a-------->                                      |
  C14 |             <------a------->                                           |
      | 54.81                      Line Plots                          435.57 |
  C14 | 1..3.12.1.131.11.1.3...1......1...1..11.1.................1            |
  C14 | ..1.1..1232....21........1.....1....1....................             |
```


Two Sample T-Test Results

	C15		C15	
Count – Mean	26	107.89	16	213.435
95% C.L. of Mean	65.71613	150.0639	−59.6476	486.5176
Std. Dev. – Std. Error	104.4225	20.47893	512.6602	128.1651

	---- Equal Variances ----		---- Unequal Variances ----	
T-Value – Prob.	−1.023283	0.3123	−0.8131928	0.4280
Degrees of Freedom		40		15.87182
Diff. – Std. Error	−105.545	103.1435	−105.545	129.7909
95% C.L. of Diff.	−314.0051	102.9151	−380.7308	169.6408

F-ratio testing group variances		24.10301	Prob. Level	0.0000

```
      | −59.6476                95% Conf. Limit Plots                 2117.22 |
  C15 |    <a>                                                                |
  C15 | <-------a----------->                                                 |
      | −59.6476                    Line Plots                       2117.22 |
  C15 | ..92622211...1..........................................             |
  C15 | ..5143.11..............................................1             |
```

Two Sample T-Test Results

	C16		C16	
Count – Mean	26	18.13346	16	18.1075
95% C.L. of Mean	15.05579	21.21114	13.6103	22.6047
Std. Dev. – Std. Error	7.620318	1.494467	8.442629	2.110657

	---- Equal Variances ----		---- Unequal Variances ----	
T-Value – Prob.	1.029187E-02	0.9918	1.003834E-02	0.9921
Degrees of Freedom		40		31.08308
Diff. – Std. Error	2.596092E-02	2.522469	2.596092E-02	2.586176
95% C.L. of Diff.	−5.07212	5.124042	−5.247818	5.299739

F-ratio testing group variances	1.227465	Prob. Level	0.3155

```
       | 1.92               95% Conf. Limit Plots              39.94|
  C16  |                      <-----a------>                        |
  C16  |                    <--------a---------->                   |
       | 1.92                    Line Plots                    39.94|
  C16  | 1..........11111..122.1212..1...31.1..1.1................1  |
  C16  | .........1...11.31111....1....1.........1....11..1........  |
```

Two Sample T-Test Results

	C17		C17	
Count – Mean	26	22.66308	16	18.14688
95% C.L. of Mean	15.92029	29.40586	9.867251	26.4265
Std. Dev. – Std. Error	16.69512	3.274183	15.54341	3.885852

	---- Equal Variances ----		---- Unequal Variances ----	
T-Value – Prob.	0.8734407	0.3876	0.8887798	0.3800
Degrees of Freedom		40		35.73254
Diff. – Std. Error	4.516201	5.170587	4.516201	5.08135
95% C.L. of Diff.	−5.933904	14.96631	−5.789525	14.82193

F-ratio testing group variances	1.153684	Prob. Level	0.3955

```
       | -14.2              95% Conf. Limit Plots              69.13|
  C17  |                      <-----a------>                        |
  C17  |                    <--------a--------->                    |
       | -14.2                   Line Plots                    69.13|
  C17  | ..1......1.1..1..121.2311...113...11..1.2................1  |
  C17  | 1......1......11.111.11....211...1..1....1...............   |
```

Two Sample T-Test Results

	C18		C18	
Count – Mean	26	5.507692	16	5.8125
95% C.L. of Mean	5.096622	5.918763	5.311339	6.313661
Std. Dev. – Std. Error	1.017811	0.1996091	0.940833	.2352082

	---- Equal Variances ----		---- Unequal Variances ----	
T-Value – Prob.	−0.969322	0.3382	−0.9880601	0.3297
Degrees of Freedom		40		35.92048
Diff. – Std. Error	−0.3048077	0.3144545	−0.3048077	0.308491
95% C.L. of Diff.	−0.9403415	0.3307262	−0.9304594	0.3208441

F-ratio testing group variances	1.170331	Prob. Level	0.3840

```
      | 3.3                    95% Conf. Limit Plots                         8 |
  C18 |                         <----a-------->                               |
  C18 |                         <-----a----------->                          |
      | 3.3                         Line Plots                              8 |
  C18 | 1.........11.1..11...2.3.1.123..111.1..1.......1.1.....1..            |
  C18 | ...........1....1.1....1.1..211.12.....1.1...1...........1            |
```


Two Sample T-Test Results

	C19		C19	
Count – Mean	26	62	16	62.93125
95% C.L. of Mean	55.18938	68.81062	54.74751	71.115
Std. Dev. – Std. Error	16.8631	3.307125	15.36341	3.840852

	---- Equal Variances ----		---- Unequal Variances ----	
T-Value – Prob.	−0.1796189	0.8584	−0.1837348	0.8553
Degrees of Freedom		40		36.29741
Diff. – Std. Error	−0.9312515	5.184596	−0.9312515	5.068453
95% C.L. of Diff.	−11.40967	9.547168	−11.21007	9.347569

F-ratio testing group variances	1.204757	Prob. Level	0.3609

```
      | 18.8                   95% Conf. Limit Plots                      91.1 |
  C19 |                         <------a-------->                             |
  C19 |                         <--------a---------->                        |
      | 18.8                        Line Plots                           91.1 |
  C19 | 1...1..........1....1..1.1..1111..1221..3211...1.....1..1             |
  C19 | ..........2...............1..111...3....11.1.11.1...1.....            |
```

Appendix F

Comparison of Values of Nineteen Variables for Merged Firms vs. Nonmerged Firms

Two Sample T-Test Results

	C1		C21	
Count – Mean	28	1.889286	29	1.861035
95% C.L. of Mean	1.050399	2.728173	1.54846	2.173609
Std. Dev. – Std. Error	2.163555	0.4088734	0.8217549	0.152596
	---- Equal Variances ----		---- Unequal Variances ----	
T-Value – Prob.	6.560463E-02	0.9479	0.0647338	0.9488
Degrees of Freedom		55		34.9483
Diff. – Std. Error	2.825117E-02	0.4306277	2.825117E-02	0.4364207
95% C.L. of Diff.	−0.8347395	0.8912419	−0.8577493	0.9142517
F-ratio testing group variances		6.931884	Prob. Level	0.0000

```
    | .08                95% Conf. Limit Plots                 8.43 |
C1  |            <------a---------->                               |
C21 |               <-a---->                                       |
    | .08                    Line Plots                       8.43 |
C1  | 2.514112..1121..11...........1..1....1.........1.........1   |
C21 | ...1.1.542..412211.1111...1..................................|
```

Two Sample T-Test Results

	C2		C22	
Count – Mean	10	0.223	22	0.7631818
95% C.L. of Mean	−1.880002E-02	0.4648	0.1735773	1.352786
Std. Dev. – Std. Error	0.3385279	0.1070519	1.329982	0.2835531

	---- Equal Variances ----		---- Unequal Variances ----	
T-Value – Prob.	−1.255551	0.2190	−1.78226	0.0860
Degrees of Freedom		30		26.80044
Diff. – Std. Error	−0.5401818	0.4302348	−0.5401818	0.3030882
95% C.L. of Diff.	−1.418829	0.3384651	−1.162235	8.187097E-02

F-ratio testing group variances		15.43485	Prob. Level	0.0001

```
     -1.880002E-02        95% Conf. Limit Plots                    6
C2   <--a---->
C22    <------a-------->
     -1.880002E-02             Line Plots                          6
C2   52.1..1...1...........................................
C22  352222..11..1......1..1................................1
```

Two Sample T-Test Results

	C3		C23	
Count – Mean	28	88.65929	29	71.41966
95% C.L. of Mean	70.29681	107.0218	62.39102	80.44829
Std. Dev. – Std. Error	47.35826	8.94987	23.73619	4.407699

	---- Equal Variances ----		---- Unequal Variances ----	
T-Value – Prob.	1.746623	0.0863	1.728046	0.0917
Degrees of Freedom		55		40.36443
Diff. – Std. Error	17.23963	9.870266	17.23963	9.976372
95% C.L. of Diff.	−2.540672	37.01994	−2.922731	37.40199

F-ratio testing group variances		3.980794	Prob. Level	0.0003

```
     8.67                95% Conf. Limit Plots               256.02
C3              <-----a------->
C23               <-a-->
     8.67                     Line Plots                     256.02
C3   1.....1.112.142..22..2.311.....12.......................1
C23  .1.....211131331214.111..11.............................
```

Two Sample T-Test Results

	C4		C24	
Count – Mean	28	7.57	29	9.583793
95% C.L. of Mean	6.086811	9.053189	7.465415	11.70217
Std. Dev. – Std. Error	3.82526	0.7229062	5.569193	1.034173

	---- Equal Variances ----		---- Unequal Variances ----	
T-Value – Prob.	−1.585786	0.1185	−1.595984	0.1167
Degrees of Freedom		55		51.31265
Diff. – Std. Error	−2.013793	1.269902	−2.013793	1.261788
95% C.L. of Diff.	−4.558714	0.5311286	−4.546551	0.5189657

F-ratio testing group variances	2.119643	Prob. Level	0.0272

```
      .97                 95% Conf. Limit Plots              20.61
C4    |                      <-----a----->                       |
C24   |                    <-------a-------->                    |
      .97                      Line Plots                   20.61
C4    |.2.....1111.121.2131111.1.1...11.1.1..1..........1........|
C24   |1.2...111..2...12.....4..11.....3...211....11......1...1.1|
```


Two Sample T-Test Results

	C5		C25	
Count – Mean	18	60.47833	29	53.93034
95% C.L. of Mean	47.40835	73.54832	17.84	90.02069
Std. Dev. – Std. Error	26.28883	6.196337	94.88114	17.61899

	---- Equal Variances ----		---- Unequal Variances ----	
T-Value – Prob.	0.2850029	0.7769	0.3505946	0.7280
Degrees of Freedom		45		34.98651
Diff. – Std. Error	6.547989	22.97517	6.547989	18.67681
95% C.L. of Diff.	−39.72574	52.82172	−31.36736	44.46334

F-ratio testing group variances	13.02619	Prob. Level	0.0000

```
      0                 95% Conf. Limit Plots              476.59
C5    |        <a--->                                           |
C25   |      <-----a------>                                     |
      0                      Line Plots                   476.59
C5    |.1.12213123.11...........................................|
C25   |63233341..1...1....................1.....................1|
```

Two Sample T-Test Results

	C6		C26	
Count – Mean	27	−2.592593E-03	28	0.7114286
95% C.L. of Mean	−0.577509	0.5723238	−22.37674	23.7996
Std. Dev. – Std. Error	1.453356	0.2796985	59.54618	11.25317

	---- Equal Variances ----		---- Unequal Variances ----	
T-Value – Prob.	−6.226848E-02	0.9506	−6.343108E-02	0.9499
Degrees of Freedom		53		27.03583
Diff. – Std. Error	−0.7140212	11.46682	−0.7140212	11.25665
95% C.L. of Diff.	−23.71335	22.2853	−23.80796	22.37992

F-ratio testing group variances		1678.664	Prob. Level	0.0000

```
       -258.07              95% Conf. Limit Plots                 138.96
C6     |                             a                                 |
C26    |                           <----a---->                         |
       -258.07                  Line Plots                        138.96
C6     |...............................................1Q..................|
C26    |1.............................................1..I411.........1......1|
```

Two Sample T-Test Results

	C7		C27	
Count – Mean	26	2.529615	29	21.15897
95% C.L. of Mean	−13.73277	18.792	13.45829	28.85964
Std. Dev. – Std. Error	40.26565	7.896743	20.245	3.759402

	---- Equal Variances ----		---- Unequal Variances ----	
T-Value – Prob.	−2.201913	0.0320	−2.130055	0.0399
Degrees of Freedom		53		36.83047
Diff. – Std. Error	−18.62935	8.46053	−18.62935	8.745951
95% C.L. of Diff.	−35.59888	−1.659821	−36.35254	−0.9061642

F-ratio testing group variances		3.955795	Prob. Level	0.0003

```
       -188.45              95% Conf. Limit Plots                  81.12
C7     |                           <--a--->                             |
C27    |                              <a->                              |
       -188.45                  Line Plots                         81.12
C7     |1...................................146912...11........         |
C27    |1...................................12625422.11.1....11         |
```

Two Sample T-Test Results

	C8		C28	
Count – Mean	28	−6.5525	29	0.6758621
95% C.L. of Mean	−11.30719	−1.797808	−12.47459	13.82632
Std. Dev. – Std. Error	12.26272	2.317436	34.57241	6.419936

	---- Equal Variances ----		---- Unequal Variances ----	
T-Value – Prob.	−1.044453	0.3008	−1.059039	0.2966
Degrees of Freedom		55		35.66597
Diff. – Std. Error	−7.228362	6.920713	−7.228362	6.8254
95% C.L. of Diff.	−21.09768	6.640952	−21.07137	6.614648

F-ratio testing group variances		7.94851	Prob. Level	0.0000

```
     | -156.71              95% Conf. Limit Plots                    66.04 |
C8   |                                         <a->                        |
C28  |                                         <--a--->                    |
     | -156.71                  Line Plots                           66.04 |
C8   | ............................111.1315452.4..............             |
C28  | 1...............................3...2215453.11.........1            |
```

Two Sample T-Test Results

	C9		C29	
Count – Mean	28	−13.285	29	−0.6768966
95% C.L. of Mean	−19.2021	−7.367904	−6.24659	4.892797
Std. Dev. – Std. Error	15.26065	2.883992	14.64267	2.719075

	---- Equal Variances ----		---- Unequal Variances ----	
T-Value – Prob.	−3.183255	0.0024	−3.180907	0.0024
Degrees of Freedom		55		56.66316
Diff. – Std. Error	−12.6081	3.960758	−12.6081	3.963682
95% C.L. of Diff.	−20.54558	−4.670627	−20.54617	−4.670032

F-ratio testing group variances		1.08619	Prob. Level	0.4141

```
     | -54.51               95% Conf. Limit Plots                    37.79 |
C9   |                      <---a----->                                    |
C29  |                       <----a------>                                 |
     | -54.51                   Line Plots                           37.79 |
C9   | ..1...1....2.....1.11.2112...321322.1......1...............          |
C29  | 1...................11.11.1..21.523342.................1            |
```

Two Sample T-Test Results

	C10		C30	
Count – Mean	28	1.064286	29	1.66069
95% C.L. of Mean	0.9003823	1.228189	1.47044	1.850939
Std. Dev. – Std. Error	0.4227198	7.988654E-02	0.5001638	9.287808E-02

	---- Equal Variances ----		---- Unequal Variances ----	
T-Value – Prob.	−4.853818	0.0000	−4.868288	0.0000
Degrees of Freedom		55		55.98024
Diff. – Std. Error	−0.596404	0.1228732	−0.596404	0.1225079
95% C.L. of Diff.	−0.8426454	−0.3501625	−0.8418161	−0.3509918

F-ratio testing group variances	1.399972	Prob. Level	0.1925

```
     |.38              95% Conf. Limit Plots                    3.37 |
C10  |           <----a---->                                         |
C30  |                   <----a----->                                |
     |.38                  Line Plots                          3.37 |
C10  |1..1113.32.131111.111.11..1...2.............................  |
C30  |...........11.111241.312.2.123.1................1........1     |
```

Two Sample T-Test Results

	C11		C31	
Count – Mean	27	80922.41	29	55555.17
95% C.L. of Mean	54688.95	107155.9	40655.61	70454.73
Std. Dev. – Std. Error	66316.68	12762.65	39170.78	7273.831

	---- Equal Variances ----		---- Unequal Variances ----	
T-Value – Prob.	1.757448	0.0845	1.726846	0.0914
Degrees of Freedom		54		42.73861
Diff. – Std. Error	25367.23	14434.13	25367.23	14689.92
95% C.L. of Diff.	−3571.518	54305.98	−4262.391	54996.86

F-ratio testing group variances	2.866297	Prob. Level	0.0038

```
     |5601             95% Conf. Limit Plots                 295437 |
C11  |          <------a------>                                      |
C31  |        <--a-->                                                |
     |5601                 Line Plots                        295437 |
C11  |122.11121.2.11..2.1.3.1...2.....1.....1..................1     |
C31  |1.222441...42.1.1..11..1..1...1............................   |
```

Two Sample T-Test Results

	C12		C32	
Count – Mean	28	16.54571	29	16.55862
95% C.L. of Mean	16.11372	16.9777	16.15186	16.96538
Std. Dev. – Std. Error	1.114133	0.2105513	1.069375	0.1985779

	---- Equal Variances ----		---- Unequal Variances ----	
T-Value – Prob.	−4.462855E-02	0.9646	−4.459589E-02	0.9646
Degrees of Freedom		55		56.66611
Diff. – Std. Error	−1.290703E-02	0.2892101	−1.290703E-02	0.2894219
95% C.L. of Diff.	−0.5924927	0.5666786	−0.5925319	0.5667179

F-ratio testing group variances		1.085461	Prob. Level	0.4147

```
        14.71                95% Conf. Limit Plots                 18.86
C12  |                       <-------a------->                          |
C32  |                       <------a------->                           |
        14.71                    Line Plots                        18.86
C12  |  1...3..11...1.111....112....1..2.2.2..21.2............1...1      |
C32  |  ..1.111..1.11.111.1.1.21.....11..31.111.12............1...1      |
```


Two Sample T-Test Results

	C13		C33	
Count – Mean	28	−61.48893	29	8.304828
95% C.L. of Mean	−109.2882	−13.68969	−5.959976	22.56963
Std. Dev. – Std. Error	123.278	23.29735	37.50202	6.96395

	---- Equal Variances ----		---- Unequal Variances ----	
T-Value – Prob.	−2.913211	0.0052	−2.870293	0.0072
Degrees of Freedom		55		32.15031
Diff. – Std. Error	−69.79376	23.95767	−69.79376	24.3159
95% C.L. of Diff.	−117.8056	−21.78187	−119.3215	−20.26603

F-ratio testing group variances		10.80592	Prob. Level	0.0000

```
       -573.94               95% Conf. Limit Plots                  140
C13  |                                      <-----a----->               |
C33  |                                              <a->                |
       -573.94                   Line Plots                         140
C13  |  1.................1.................11.12212724111........        |
C33  |  .....................................1.332575..2.....1          |
```

Two Sample T-Test Results

	C14		C34	
Count – Mean	28	155.2568	29	195.4465
95% C.L. of Mean	121.789	188.7246	173.8463	217.0468
Std. Dev. – Std. Error	86.31598	16.31219	56.78689	10.54506

	---- Equal Variances ----		---- Unequal Variances ----	
T-Value – Prob.	−2.083778	0.0418	−2.069094	0.0439
Degrees of Freedom		55		47.88182
Diff. – Std. Error	−40.18976	19.28697	−40.18976	19.42384
95% C.L. of Diff.	−78.84141	−1.538109	−79.2439	−1.135612

F-ratio testing group variances		2.310395	Prob. Level	0.0157

```
      43.92                95% Conf. Limit Plots              449.46
C14 |              <------a----->                                  |
C34 |                   <----a---->                                |
      43.92                   Line Plots                     449.46
C14 | 1..111321.1.12221...2.....14.......1....................1    |
C34 | ........21...21..123122231.2.2.1................1........     |
```

Two Sample T-Test Results

	C15		C35	
Count – Mean	28	211.095	29	2340.254
95% C.L. of Mean	27.26215	394.9279	−2154.804	6835.313
Std. Dev. – Std. Error	474.1192	89.60011	11817.46	2194.448

	---- Equal Variances ----		---- Unequal Variances ----	
T-Value – Prob.	−0.9523357	0.3451	−0.9694407	0.3406
Degrees of Freedom		55		28.10002
Diff. – Std. Error	−2129.159	2235.723	−2129.159	2196.276
95% C.L. of Diff.	−6609.615	2351.296	−6627.774	2369.456

F-ratio testing group variances		621.2599	Prob. Level	0.0000

```
     -2154.804            95% Conf. Limit Plots              63774
C15 | a                                                          |
C35 | <-----a------>                                             |
     -2154.804                Line Plots                    63774
C15 | .1N4.......................................................|
C35 | ..R1......................................................1|
```

Two Sample T-Test Results

	C16		C36	
Count – Mean	28	46.31179	29	31.13724
95% C.L. of Mean	30.68024	61.94333	24.39515	37.87934
Std. Dev. – Std. Error	40.31496	7.618813	17.7249	3.291431

	---- Equal Variances ----		---- Unequal Variances ----	
T-Value – Prob.	1.850612	0.0696	1.828393	0.0753
Degrees of Freedom		55		37.50483
Diff. – Std. Error	15.17455	8.199742	15.17455	8.299387
95% C.L. of Diff.	−1.25798	31.60707	−1.627222	31.97631

F-ratio testing group variances	5.173269	Prob. Level	0.0000

```
       5.79              95% Conf. Limit Plots              161.43 |
C16 |              <--------a-------->
C36 |            <-a-->
       5.79                 Line Plots                      161.43 |
C16 | 211.111134.23.1..1..........1...1........2...1.............1
C36 | ..4.134223.121111.1.1..........1.........................
```

Two Sample T-Test Results

	C17		C37	
Count – Mean	28	−7.162143	29	16.57241
95% C.L. of Mean	−22.93649	8.612203	10.65484	22.48999
Std. Dev. – Std. Error	40.68326	7.688414	15.55725	2.888909

	---- Equal Variances ----		---- Unequal Variances ----	
T-Value – Prob.	−2.928506	0.0049	−2.889788	0.0066
Degrees of Freedom		55		35.05293
Diff. – Std. Error	−23.73456	8.104665	−23.73456	8.213252
95% C.L. of Diff.	−39.97655	−7.492571	−40.40701	−7.062113

F-ratio testing group variances	6.838581	Prob. Level	0.0000

```
      -105.04             95% Conf. Limit Plots              66.67 |
C17 |              <--------a-------->
C37 |                     <-a->
      -105.04                Line Plots                       66.67 |
C17 | 1..1....1..........1...1.21.1..231..21.2.12..11.1...1....1
C37 | ...........................2......422232312122....1.....
```

Two Sample T-Test Results

	C18		C38	
Count – Mean	28	10.3	29	12.82069
95% C.L. of Mean	7.781477	12.81852	3.376746	22.26463
Std. Dev. – Std. Error	6.495469	1.227528	24.82803	4.610449

	---- Equal Variances ----		---- Unequal Variances ----	
T-Value – Prob.	−0.5201653	0.6050	−0.5283283	0.6609
Degrees of Freedom		55		32.22615
Diff. – Std. Error	−2.520689	4.845938	−2.520689	4.771066
95% C.L. of Diff.	−12.23209	7.190714	−12.23843	7.197047

F-ratio testing group variances		14.61045	Prob. Level	0.0000

```
     2.7                95% Conf. Limit Plots                 135.5
C18 |    <a>                                                       |
C38 | <-----a----->                                                |
     2.7                    Line Plots                        135.5
C18 | 1A51,42221...........................................        |
C38 | 2H2131..1.........1........................................1 |
```

Two Sample T-Test Results

	C19		C39	
Count – Mean	28	44.99643	29	53.65862
95% C.L. of Mean	37.78237	52.21049	46.94577	60.37147
Std. Dev. – Std. Error	18.60562	3.516132	17.64802	3.277154

	---- Equal Variances ----		---- Unequal Variances ----	
T-Value – Prob.	−1.803864	0.0767	−1.802163	0.0768
Degrees of Freedom		55		56.55444
Diff. – Std. Error	−8.66219	4.80202	−8.66219	4.806551
95% C.L. of Diff.	−18.28558	.9612007	−18.28867	0.9642859

F-ratio testing group variances		1.111467	Prob. Level	0.3909

```
     13.3               95% Conf. Limit Plots                  99.3
C19 |                    <------a------>                            |
C39 |                    <------a----->                            |
     13.3                   Line Plots                         99.3
C19 | 1..1.11.2...21.22.1..1.12..1.2....13....111...............    |
C39 | ...........2311..1121.1..112.21.21..11...2.....1........1     |
```

Bibliography

Government Publications

___ *Individual Hospital Financial Data for California June 30, 1979-June 29, 1990*. Sacramento, CA: Office of Statewide Health Planning and Development, June 1980-1991.

Books

Hair, Joseph F., Rolph E. Anderson, and Ronald L. Tatham. *Multivariate Data Analysis: With Readings*. New York: Macmillan Publishing Company, 1987.

Merwin, Charles. *Financing Small Corporations in Five Manufacturing Industries: 1926-32*. Bureau of Economic Research: New York, 1942.

Mullner, Ross M. and Ronald M. Anderson. "A Descriptive and Financial Ratio Analysis of Merged and Consolidated Hospitals: United States 1980-1985." In *Advances in Health Economics and Health Services Research*, edited by Richard M. Scheffler and Louis F. Rossiter. Greenwich, CT: Jai Press, 1987.

Singh, Ajit. *Takeovers: Their Relevance to the Stock Market and the Theory of the Firm*. Cambridge: Cambridge University Press, 1971.

Smith, Raymond A. and Arthur H. Winakor. *Changes in the Financial Structure of Unsuccessful Industrial Corporations*. Bureau of Business Research, University of Illinois, 1935.

Dissertations

Lin, You-an Robert. "The Use of Supplementing Accounting Disclosures for Corporate Takeover Targets Prediction." PhD diss., University of California, Los Angeles, 1989.

Omurtak, Sehrazat Saridereli. "Financial Ratios as Predictors of Corporate Acquisition Candidates by Industry." PhD diss., University of Missouri, Rolla, 1986.

Treat, Thomas Frank. "A Study of the Characteristics and Performance of Merged Hospitals in the United States." PhD diss., Texas A&M University, 1973.

Periodicals

Mergers and Acquisitions, May/June 1991-1984.

Mergers and Acquisitions, May/June 1992.

Altman, Edward I. "Financial Ratios, Discriminant Analysis, and the Prediction of Corporate Bankruptcy." *The Journal of Finance*, September 1968, 589-609.

Anders, George. "Health Care Firms Face Checkup for Merger Potential." *The Wall Street Journal*, October 12, 1993, B1, B6.

Beaver, William F. "Financial Ratios as Predictors of Failure." *Empirical Research in Accounting: Selected Studies, 1966*. Institute of Professional Accounting, Graduate School of Business (University of Chicago, 1967), 71-111.

Beaver, William H., John W. Kennelly, and William M. Voss. "Predictive Ability as a Criterion for the Evaluation of Accounting Data." *The Accounting Review*, October 1968, 675-683.

Belkaoui, Ahmed. "Financial Ratios as Predictors of Canadian Takeovers." *Journal of Business Finance & Accounting*, Spring 1978, 93-107.

Bruno, Albert V., Joel K. Leidecker, and Carol G. Torgrimson. "Sizing Up Your Company's Takeover Vulnerability." *Mergers and Acquisitions*, Summer 1985, 42-49.

Cherskov, Myk. "What's Driving Upcoming Mergers?" *Hospitals*, January 5, 1987, 36-40.

Cleverley, William O. "Financial Ratios: Summary Indicators for Management Decision Making." *Hospital & Health Services Administration*, Special 1, 1981, 26-47.

Fisher, May Jane. "Health Care Costs in 2000 Seen at 'Staggering' $1.5 Trillion." *National Underwriter*, November 12, 1990, 1-26.

Fisher, R. A. "The Use of Multiple Measurements in Taxonomic Problems." *Annals of Eugenics*, September 1936, 179-188.

Fitzpatrick, Paul J. "A Comparison of the Ratios of Successful Industrial Enterprises with Those of Failed Companies." *The Certified Public Accountant*, October 1932, 598-605.

Geisel, Jerry. "Health Costs More Than Doubled in 1980s." *Business Insurance*, May 21, 1990, 15.

Gort, Michael. "An Economic Disturbance Theory of Mergers." *Quarterly Journal of Economics*, November 1969, 624-659.

Grant, Edward A. and Edward J. Giniat. "Evaluating Mergers and Acquisitions with a Purchase Investigation." *Healthcare Financial Management*, April 1988, 72-82.

Greene, Jay. "The Costs of Hospital Mergers." *Modern Healthcare*, February 3, 1992, 36-43.

Hise, Richard J. "Evaluating Marketing Assets in Mergers and Acquisitions." *The Journal of Business Strategy*, July/August 1991, 46-51.

Ijiri, Yuji and Robert K. Jaedicke. "Reliability and Objectivity of Accounting Measurements." *The Accounting Review*, July 1966, 474-483.

Levitz, Gary S. and Paul P. Brooke Jr. "Independent versus System-Affiliated Hospitals: A Comparative Analysis of Financial Performance, Cost and Productivity." *Health Services Research*, August 1985, 315-339.

Lewellyn, Wilbur G. "A Pure Financial Rationale for the Conglomerate Merger." *The Journal of Finance*, May 1971, 521-537.

McCue, Michael J., Tom McCue, and John R. C. Wheeler. "An Assessment of Hospital Acquisition Prices." *Inquiry*, Summer 1988, 290-296.

Melicher, Ronald W. and James F. Neilsen. "Financial Factors That Affect Acquisition Prices." *Review of Business & Economic Research*, Winter 1977/8, 95-106.

Merjos, Anna. "Takeover Targets," *Barrons*, May 15, 1978, 9-35 (interrupted).

Mueller, Dennis C. "A Theory of Conglomerate Mergers." *Quarterly Journal of Economics*, November 1969, 643-659.

Nielsen, James F. and Ronald W. Melicher. "A Financial Analysis of Acquisition and Merger Premiums." *Journal of Financial and Quantitative Analysis*, March 1973, 139-148.

Palepu, Krishna G. "Predicting Takeover Targets." *Journal of Accounting and Economics*, March 1986, 3-35.

Palm, Kari Super. "Half of CEOs in Survey See Their Hospital Included in a Transition Within 5 Years." *Modern Healthcare*, June 10, 1988, 40-42.

Rich, Spencer. "Health Costs to Consume 16% of GNP by 2000, Agency Says." *The Washington Post*, August 24, 1991, p. A2.

Rosendale, William M. "Credit Department Methods." *The Bankers Magazine*, 1908, 183-194.

Shrieves, Ronald E. and Donald L. Stevens. "Bankruptcy Avoidance as a Motive for Merger." *Journal of Financial and Quantitative Analysis*, September 1979, 501-515.

Simkowitz, Michael and Robert J. Monroe. "A Discriminant Analysis Function for Conglomerate Targets." *The Southern Journal of Business*, November 1971, 1-16.

Skrzycki, Cindy. "Cost of Medical Benefits Said to Rise 21% a Year." *The Washington Post*, January 19, 1991, E5.

Stevens, Donald L. "Financial Characteristics of Merged Firms: A Multivariate Analysis." *Journal of Financial and Quantitative Analysis*, March 1973, 149-158.

Taussig, Russell A. and Samuel L. Hayes III. "Cash Take-Overs and Accounting Valuations." *The Accounting Review*, January 1968, 68-74.

Vance, Jack O. "Is Your Company a Takeover Target?" *Harvard Business Review*, May-June 1969, 95-98.

Wansley, James W. "Discriminant Analysis and Merger Theory." *Review of Business & Economic Research*, Fall 1984, 76-85.

Wansley, James W., and William R. Lane. "A Financial Profile of Merged Firms." *Review of Business & Economic Research*, Fall 1984, 87-98.

Index

Page numbers followed by the letter "f" indicate figures; those followed by the letter "t" indicate tables.

T - #0587 - 101024 - C0 - 212/152/8 - PB - 9780789001825 - Gloss Lamination